DIS(

MW01298368

TABLE OF CONTENTS

THE BEGINNING

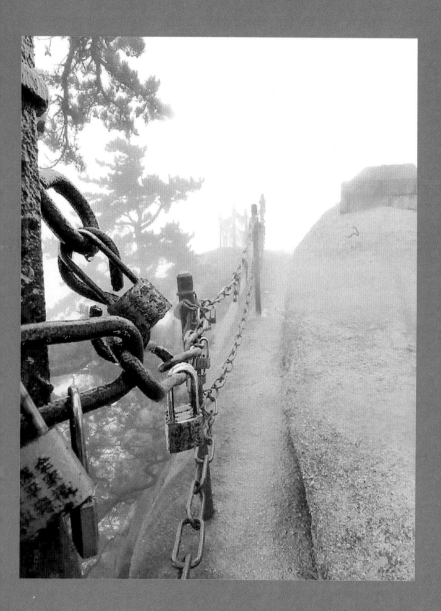

The greatest advantage of The *Laws of Aesthetics* is that the book goes beyond the mere physical level and also addresses the psychological and environmental factors that contribute to and often determine your ability to achieve fat loss and perfect abs.

From fat loss secrets to ideal fat loss nutrition, workout, and supplement programs, The *Laws of Aesthetics* puts it all together for you in an easy and entertaining read.

You'll be provided with a step-by-step outline of exactly what you need to do to drop as much body fat as necessary and attain the best-looking abs and body possible.

This book is also associated with a support website featuring instructional videos and helpful tips to enhance your understanding of the information provided here.

To enhance your learning, this book comes with free video instruction. Please email me a receipt of your purchase at **etrufkin@gmail.com** After I receive a picture of your receipt, you will be provided access to the video content.

The problem with fitness books is that they mislead you into believing that working out is the most important variable when it comes to your health, your physical fitness, and your quest for perfect abs. In truth, working out is one of the *least* important variables in any training routine. It's important to understand that fitness is built upon a hierarchy of needs. Fundamental needs must to be met before progressing to other, more advanced needs. A successful fitness program can be more accurately understood by considering the following pyramid:

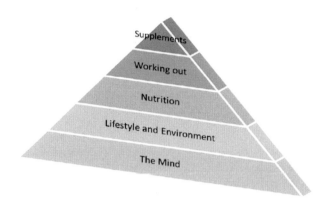

As you can see from the picture above, THE MIND, which accounts for your motivation, lays the foundation for any fitness program. THE MIND is the single most important variable in any training routine. Without a solid mindset that sustains consistent motivation levels, you simply will not train—and your body won't change, no matter how many gym memberships or fat loss pills you buy, or how many fitness books you read. Being and staying motivated is actually the most important variable in any training routine. If this variable breaks down or doesn't exist to begin with, the entire pyramid will crumble.

For most people, finding and keeping the motivation to train and, more importantly, continue training is the most challenging aspect of any training routine. Everyone in America has access to a gym these days. There is more information available on fitness and nutrition than ever before. Why is it that Americans keep getting fatter (and uglier)? It's not the processed food--there is plenty of healthy food out there too. It's certainly not due to a lack of gyms. Rather, lack of motivation to train is the answer. Most Americans are just not terribly motivated to work out, eat right, or do all the other things that healthy living requires. And if people do get motivated to train, they don't stay motivated for prolonged periods of time.

Don't get me wrong, I'm not saying that we are not motivated in general. Americans are some of the hardest-working people I've ever met. It's just that most Americans lack motivation when it comes to working out, dropping body fat, and achieving the best-looking body they possibly can.

Just remember, you must stay motivated in order to stay consistent with training. And this is why the mind lays the foundation for any training routine or fitness journey, and is the single most important variable that will determine success.

After understanding the importance of mind and motivation, the next step is to understand the importance of lifestyle and environment and how they tie into a fitness program. Just like any other endeavor, training requires an optimal environment and lifestyle in order to enhance your results and allow you to continue training for any length of time, or indeed indefinitely.

To address this step a little better, let us talk about the New Year resolution fitness crowd. The biggest mistake the New Year's crowd makes when starting a fitness program is investing all their time and energy into working out, believing that more workouts are the solution to their problem. However, the factors that led them to be inconsistent and unhealthy to begin with were certain lifestyle patterns, sustained over long periods of time, that lead to inconsistent exercise patterns and eating habits. Attempts at regular exercise within the constraints of their old lifestyle inevitably lead to skipping one workout, then two, then three, then a week here and there, until one day they look back and they haven't trained for months… or years. Thus, without fixing those same lifestyle patterns that led them to be inconsistent in the past, there is little point in starting a training routine or even a nutrition program in the present or future. If they do start a nutrition program or workout program without addressing the lifestyle and environmental variable, they will simply fall back into their old patterns of inconsistency, just like 99.9% of New Year resolution gym goers.

Now, if you are motivated and have the right lifestyle and environment to enhance the training process, it's time to concentrate on getting your nutrition in check. Again, while the most important variable is the mind and the second is lifestyle and environment, the third is nutrition. Only once you've figured out a way to stay motivated and established ideal lifestyle patterns should you begin a nutrition program. Nutrition is far more important than working out itself, especially if you want to achieve ripped abs and an ultra low body fat percentage. Working out for hours on end will not do anything for you if you're getting wasted on the weekends, staying out late several nights a week, and eating junk food even once or twice a week. In terms of fat loss and weight reduction, you could get far better results by following a nutrition program 100% without working out at all, than by working out intensively and eating poorly. Keep that in mind.

After learning how to keep motivated, understanding and establishing the proper lifestyle and environment, and following a nutrition program –then and only then should one begin a workout program. It is tempting to rush into the workout program first, but you must not do this, because if you do not address the other issues you will be inconsistent with your training and will thus be consistently out of shape. You will begin a training routine and quit within weeks. You will eat well for a little while but soon return to your old ways. If you want to be consistent, without falling back into inconsistency, if you want to be truly successful long term, to develop the best-looking body possible and to sustain that picture-perfect body over a long period of time, you must master the other variables before beginning a workout program. Following a workout program consistently will also be much easier when all the other aspects are addressed first.

As you can see, then, working out is one of the less important variables in any workout routine. It's definitely important, because everything in the pyramid is important, but it is nothing if the foundation blocks of mind, lifestyle, environment and nutrition are not in place. You must master these first fundamental variables before moving on to the workout program.

Supplements comprise the very peak of the pyramid, but this fact does not make them the most important variable—far from it. Rather, supplements are at the top to indicate that unless all the other variables are in place, supplements will accomplish nothing and are a complete waste of money.

HOW TO USE THIS BOOK

Read the chapters of this book sequentially. The chapters will explain all the points I've covered in the introduction in great detail and clarify how you can apply the information directly. You'll learn how to adopt a strong mindset and how to engineer the ideal lifestyle to optimize your fitness goals and keep yourself consistent. You'll also be provided with an ideal fat loss workout, nutrition and supplement program. On top of that, you'll also find a chapter on fat loss trickery -- something I've created for people who have a particularly tough time losing body fat and achieving their ideal body type.

Most importantly, make sure to take consistent action based on all the advice provided within this book. If you do not work, the information in this book will not work for you.

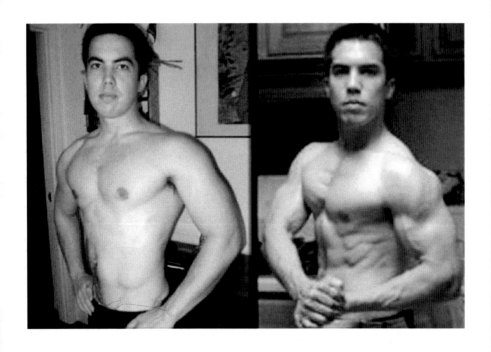

KYLE NAGAO

THE MIND

"MINDSET"

A set of beliefs or a way of thinking that determines one's behavior and outlook.

1

I get a lot of people who come in for training and ask, over and over again, how to develop the perfect body. They ask about specific supplements, specific workouts, and/or specific things to eat, hoping to find the secret in those three categories. What they fail to realize is that, although the knowledge of supplements, nutrition, and training are important, THE MOST important tool of all in the process of developing a perfect body is the MIND.

It is vital to understand that the mind is the one stumbling block that prevents 99% of people from accomplishing their goals in life. It is the mind that determines whether you will or will not accomplish difficult goals. It is the mind that makes you work out with killer intensity until you can't even walk out of the gym. It is the mind that makes you work out 2 to 3 hours a day when you could be doing other things, like socializing. It is the mind that visualizes how a body should look, how your day should look to optimize the development of your physique, and what type of friends you should make to help facilitate your pursuit of a perfect body. It is the mind that separates a winner from a loser, a person that has done something with their life from a person that has done nothing with their life--and it is the mind that composes intelligent workout, nutrition, and supplement programs to make all your fitness objectives become reality. You must train your mind, because it is your mind that tells your body to train.

Once people realize that the mind is more important than any training routine, supplement or fancy gym, they will be far more successful at attaining their goals. You must train your mind to work to your advantage, instead of your disadvantage.

How do I know if I have a strong mindset?

I believe there are four key traits that determine if a person is going to be successful in seeing their fitness goals through. If one of these mental traits is missing, a person will not be able to see their goals through.

First Key Mental Trait: DESIRE

You have to want a perfect body. The desire lays a blueprint for you to achieve a perfect body.

Second Key Mental Trait: EMOTIONAL RESPONSE

The thought of having a perfect body must trigger a genuine, positive emotional response within you. You should feel great just thinking about having a perfect body—and even better when you think about the process of accomplishing it. If this positive emotional reaction is absent, you will not be able to muster the enthusiasm and drive needed to realize your goal—long term.

Third Key Mental Trait: SELF-BELIEF

The thought of having a perfect body must trigger a genuine, positive You must have a strong belief that your desire will come true. You must have confidence in yourself that with enough work, enough knowledge, and enough patience, you can do it. There should be no doubt in your mind that you will have a perfect body—that it's only a matter of time. If you have any doubt whatsoever, this doubt will creep into your plans of attaining a perfect body and will sabotage you. There must be NO doubt that your desire will come true.

Fourth Key Mental Trait: COMPULSIVE FOCUS ON DESIRE

Finding yourself compulsively thinking about getting and maintaining the perfect body and every-thing that goes with it is a sign that you have the fourth key mental trait: compulsive focus on that desire for the perfect body. Once nothing else in life seems to matter as much as achieving the perfect body, your thoughts are strongly aligned with your desire of having a perfect body and you have an exponentially greater chance of seeing your desire through.

Here's an example of daily thought patterns for a person
who sees minimal results:

2 hours thinking about Facebook and other similar subjects, 2 hours spent attending mentally to TV watching, 8-12 hours attending to work matters, and 1 hour spent to attaining a ripped physique.

Notice how scattered and widely distributed this person's thought patterns are. He spends his day thinking about a million different things, most of which have nothing to do with his goal of achieving a perfect body. This person is definitely busy, but he's busy doing all the wrong stuff--doing things which, for the most part, get him absolutely no closer to achieving his goal. For instance, out of the 24 hours available in a day, this person only spends one hour attending to his goal of being ripped. With so little time spent focusing on that goal, naturally, only minimal results can be expected in return.

Now let's consider the example of a very dedicated
person's daily thought patterns:

Getting ripped and what it takes to facilitate that process is all this guy thinks about. The dedicated person spends most, if not all of his time concentrating on his desire. He is just as busy during the day as the "typical person" mentioned above, but this person's actions and thoughts are always working to bring him closer to achieving his goal. They are always aligned with his goal of being ripped.

What do your current thought patterns look like?
How do you need to change to quickly turn your desire into reality?

The formula for a strong mindset that will result in the perfect body:

Desire + emotional response + confidence + compulsive focus on that desire
=
Strong mindset and high likelihood of completing a goal

It is impossible to overstate the importance of the four key points above. If even one of those key traits is absent, you will not succeed.

Once that strong mindset is in place, there are a few other mental traits that determine if someone will succeed or not.

AN ABILITY TO EXERT STRONG CONTROL OVER YOUR EMOTIONS—ALSO KNOWN AS

Discipline:

You're going to need to learn to conquer your emotions. If you want to succeed, they simply have to be controlled and managed. Your emotions have to work for you, not against you. People that are successful or masters at anything are masters at controlling their emotions. This one is tough-- because people are naturally hedonistic creatures. They want to have fun, have sex, and do things that don't require much consideration or elaborate thought and effort. However, if you want to develop the most aesthetically appealing body out there, *you have to learn to control your emotions or they will control you.* It's as simple as that. Emotions are like the wind-- they blow in all sorts of directions. You can't allow your dream of developing a perfect body to be blown off course because of *petty emotions.* Make decisions for yourself. Don't allow emotions to make them for you.

I call emotions "the voice inside your head". Whenever times get hard—whenever they get really, really hard—that voice will start trying to talk you out of doing something you initially intended and wanted to do. Most people listen to the voice. That's why most people never end up seeing through their dreams in life. *The voice is the ultimate killer of dreams.* It's pathetic. The voice will throw apparently logical arguments your way, arguments that totally make sense at the time. The voice will tell you that life is short, that you are young, that you should drop your studies or work responsibilities and go to that party. Honestly, the voice often has a point—from its hedonistic perspective, that is. But although the voice is right about how to temporarily satisfy hedonistic desires, it couldn't be more wrong when it comes to seeing goals through—long term.

Positive thinking:

Training yourself to be genuinely more positive in life will bring you more happiness and joy than any amount of money or material possessions. Life is all about perception. In addition, once you start training your mind to think positively, you'll begin to see opportunities where most people would see setbacks and problems.

If this is an area you feel you need to work on, checkout the following sources:

www.journeysofwisdom.com
How to Find and Live Your Legacy Live: PPS Lesson 1 with Paul Chek

The material is deep—but they will provide you with tools that will help you identify your path in life as well as your core values. Once you're on the right path for you, you will automatically become way more positive—and happier too.

Don't limit your thinking and potential:

Train your mind to always think big and attempt the impossible. Don't just ask to lose 5lbs of fat and look better for a party, because aiming low will cause you to hit low. Rather, seek to be the most shredded human being on the planet with perfect symmetry and muscle development. Don't just think in terms of being a good-looking guy; instead, seek to be the Best-looking guy in town. The idea here is that even if you aim impossibly high and fall short, you will still do better than if you aim low and hit the mark.

Learning to control the direction of your thoughts:

Most people have scattered thinking patterns. Their thoughts come and go almost at random all day long. They lack focus--there is no congruency in their thinking. One second they could be thinking about Facebook, then the next moment their thoughts turn to a person they want to date, and an hour later their attention will have flitted to something else. People who think this way generally don't accomplish much, because they don't set their mind to any one thing. If you are plagued with this type of thinking, you must learn to direct your thoughts in a way that will benefit the realization of your desire. You have to train yourself to focus intensely on your desire and on every factor that can help facilitate the achievement of what you desire.

Here are some ways to do this:
Note Card Trick: This is a powerful and easily implemented tool that can help direct your thoughts and keep you focused on your goal. Purchase some note cards. Now, write on the note cards what you're trying to achieve. For best results place a note card in the glove compartment of your car, right next to your bed, and on your bathroom mirror and office table. Every time you walk past the card, force yourself to read the goals you have written on them.
Notebook Trick: The notebook can be treated as a kind of diary. In this notebook, you want to write what you're trying to achieve and how you plan to go about achieving it. Just by writing this down, you will increase your focus and memory retention tremendously and thus will be more likely to remember your goals throughout each day, giving them more weight in your decision-making process, which enhances your ability to see them through.
Voice Recorder Trick: This is probably one of the most powerful tools for directing your thoughts and keeping you focused on your goal. Write out on paper what you're trying to achieve. Now, record yourself reading aloud what you have written.
For overall best results, I advise you to implement all three of these techniques on a consistent basis. If you have a history of not seeing goals through, I would recommend you implement them right away. Not only will they remind you to focus solely on your goal, but they will also increase your confidence and willingness to see goals through.

Problem-solving oriented thinking:

Think about the solution instead of the problem. Many people only think about their problems, whereas successful people are in the habit of focusing on the solutions to their problems, instead of the problems themselves.

Here is a typical thought pattern of a non-successful person:
I'm fat. I hate being fat. Being fat hurts my social life. Naturally, the result is that the person becomes depressed and demoralized.

Here is a typical thought pattern of a successful person:
If I'm going to be in shape, I need to educate myself about nutrition and learn to stabilize my emotions. I'll go buy a book on nutrition and human motivation.
This person doesn't even think about his problem, but rather focuses on the next step— he spends all his time thinking about a solution to the problem, and most importantly, he takes ACTION! The result is that this person accomplishes his goal of losing weight. You will fail at times. Learn from your failure and continue to take action.

You must be able to develop the means to take you to the next level

You need to figure out what motivates you in life. What gives you enough energy to accomplish anything and everything you set out to accomplish. Basically, you need to find your legacy, your path, your true meaning in life. Once that is found, you will have infinite motivation. It's foolish to train yourself to be motivated to do something you're not destined to do in this universe. You don't need motivation. You need a life path. If you feel you're lacking in this area, check out the material I listed on page 11. It will provide you with the tools necessary to begin taking action and start figuring out your legacy.

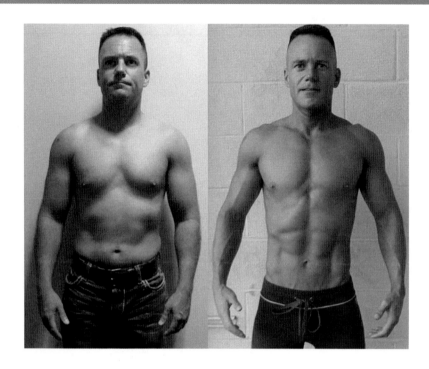

RON NORLIN

ENGINEERING YOUR LIFESTYLE

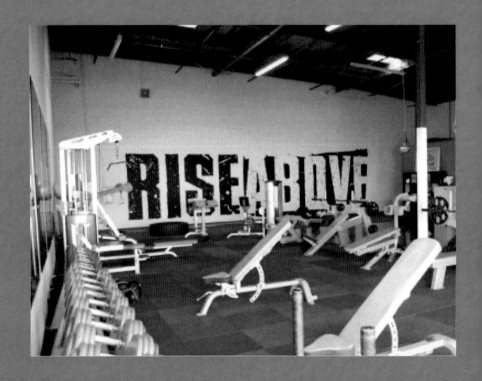

2

Once you have established the right mindset—which, once again, lays the foundation for any training routine and largely determines whether you're going to see your goal through--you still have to contend with lifestyle and environmental factors. These factors play a major role in your journey. Here are some key variables to consider and possibly modify to optimize your results:

A room built for success:

The first place you need to start is your room. Your living space is important because it's the first thing you see upon waking up, and the last thing you see before going to bed. To get the most out of a training program, you need to optimize your room to attain your goal of a perfect body. Here are some key ways to do so:

The vision board:

If you have trouble seeing long term goals through, a vision board might be the solution. A vision board is basically a collection of images of things a person is trying to achieve and what they want to have in life.

Here is what you need to do:

Step 1: Purchase a paper board at your local Wal-Mart or Target. At home, search online or in magazines for pictures representing your idea of a perfect body, as well as pictures illustrating anything you associate with having a perfect body and enjoying perfect health. These benefits might include getting positive attention, having your pick of romantic partners, or being generally perceived as more attractive; thus, you might look for images of beautiful, healthy people enjoying their health and fitness, gym pictures, pictures of attractive people with perfect skin or hair, pictures of ideal looking body parts such as chest, arms, shoulder, abs, etc. Cut these pictures out or print them out, and glue them on this board. Make it into a huge collage.

Step 2: Once you're finished with your vision board, you need to create a strategy for how to achieve that vision. This is called the Strategy Board. Don't worry--I know you probably don't know how to attain the perfect body yet... that's why you bought this book! However, I will soon outline that strategy for you here, so all you will need to do is depict it.

For the strategy board, buy a dry erase board and a few dry markers. (Yes, all these boards will cost a little bit of money, but consider it an investment in making yourself a better person and improving your quality of life.) When you work on improving yourself, you never lose.

Step 3: Place this board in the most visible portion of your room so that when you wake up, the board will be the first thing you see every single morning. If you look at this board first thing in the morning, all of your thoughts and actions that day will be primed to accomplish your goal. The board is also the last thing you're going to see before going to bed, once again reminding you of all of your goals. Ensuring constant awareness of your goals and providing yourself with constant reminders of these goals is a great way to consistently see your plans through. Implement this strategy and you will quickly notice that you are accomplishing many more of your objectives.

Role model board:

Having role models who are, one way or another, aligned with your desires in life is another way to see goals through and accomplish everything you want to accomplish. Your role models should represent positive traits such as discipline, hard work, integrity, fearlessness, strength of character etc. Having pictures of these people in your room will remind you every day of the person you want to and need to become in order to achieve your desires.

Weekly calendar:

A weekly calendar is an outline of exactly what needs to be done every single day during the week. Planning everything a week in advance and having the discipline to carry out that planning provides a sure path to success. Every single successful person in the world does this to a certain extent, and so should you if you want to be successful. Beyond increasing your efficiency and productivity during the week, another tremendous benefit of having a weekly calendar is decreasing your stress levels. By being more organized and purpose-driven during the week, you will feel less scattered in your thoughts and actions, and you will therefore experience far less stress. Also, train yourself to perceive these weekly calendars as contracts that you're obligated to accomplish no matter what--and really hold yourself accountable for fulfilling these contracts.

Once again, you really must have the discipline and maturity to religiously follow your weekly calendar. You also have to get in the habit of doing and thinking about ONE ACTIVITY at a time. What I mean by this is that when you're at your job, you should be thinking about nothing but your job. When you're working out, you want to be 100% absorbed in the workout, mentally and physically – not checking your phone, carrying on a conversation or watching the latest sporting event. You need to teach yourself to be 100% focused, mentally and physically, on one activity at a time.

Most people try to do far too many things at once, or allow themselves to be constantly distracted even as they are trying to accomplish something. Everyone knows that guy at the gym … the one who is endlessly walking around, chatting to people around him, or checking Facebook or his phone. Has his body changed at all in the last couple of years?

No. Why?

He hasn't mastered the art of concentrated effort. Or what about that friend who is always talking about achieving this and that? It sounds impressive, and he certainly seems to have big plans--but for some reason he never achieves anything noteworthy. Well, the reason he doesn't achieve anything is because he hasn't mastered the art of concentrated effort, among other problems.

How to Have More Time for Workouts and Less Stress During the Week:
I see so many people who keep themselves terribly busy throughout the day with stuff that gets them nowhere closer to where they want to be in life. They are doing things that keep them busy, take up their time, take up their energy, and increase their stress, but in NO SHAPE OR FORM help them make any headway with their most important goals. Year after year flies by and they ask themselves why they're so busy, but never progressing in life -- just getting busier.

It's a mystery to them… but it shouldn't be.

Here is what you need to do to separate yourself from the aimless zombie crowd:
Step 1: First and foremost, get rid of Facebook, MySpace, Twitter, and any other social media website you have. Your life would be a lot more interesting if you spent less of your free time on that nonsense and more of your free time actually doing cool stuff. By getting rid of these sites, you not only free up your time, but you also have one less thing to check and worry about on a day-to-day basis. This will align your thought patterns more closely with your goals,

you'll become more socially active in real life, and you'll feel less overwhelmed during the day. This will lead to less stress and more energy. Stress is a massive energy drain, so anything you can do to decrease stress, no matter how small, will lead to more energy.

Step 2:   Second, leave your personal phone in the car when you go to work, and only check it during lunch and when you get off work. I personally only check my phone during lunch time. Unless you're the president of the United States, there is no reason whatsoever to be on standby waiting to respond to every single text, voicemail, and email on the dot.

Step 3:   Personal email, just like cell phone use, needs to be limited throughout the day for all the same reasons listed in point 2.

Step 4:   Don't watch the news on TV. Ever. I mean it. Daily news in America is hopelessly negative,, inaccurate, and can only cause you to feel down. 99% of broadcasts and stories are about people facing hopeless problems, tragedy, petty gossip and other negative subject material. The worst thing you can do is to watch the news first thing in the morning. Talk about programming your brain with negative thoughts right from the get-go! One morning in college, when I was having breakfast with a couple of fellow students, I noticed that the news was playing in the background and that the conversations at the table tended to be negative. The next morning, I turned off the TV before anyone got to the cafeteria and started a conversation on a positive note. All of a sudden, everyone was talking about positive things at the table. Many scientific studies on human behavior can objectively confirm this common-sense observation. Bottom line: don't watch the news.

And no, you're not an uninformed and irresponsible citizen just because you don't watch the news—most of the TV news we watch is without meaningful content anyway, diluted and exaggerated.

Step 5:   In fact, if you're seriously dedicated about getting the most out of life, just stop watching TV all together. I was never a big TV watcher, but after college I quit cold turkey. I don't even own a TV anymore. All of a sudden I had 4-5 extra hours per week to do other, more productive things, like learn how to dance, take classes on how to be a better public speaker, and other stuff that has helped me far more than anything I could possibly get from watching TV. Also, people tend to watch TV when they have nothing to do. Since they're already in an idle and passive state, their brain is especially receptive to any information they happen to be watching at any given moment. If you watch the news, which spits out negative trash left and right, you'll think negatively. If you watch reality TV shows that are filled with aimless, selfish attention seekers, you'll be more likely to emulate that lifestyle and become like them (please don't).

The general idea here is: if it doesn't relate to your goal, simply don't give it your attention or your energy. You really have to train yourself to be selective about the information your brain takes in on a daily basis.

Let us take a look at a chart that exhibits how much less stressful a person's day is when it's not overloaded with useless information and petty, unproductive tasks:

As you can see, Person B, who is not on information overload, is clearly less stressed, and has more available time throughout the day. You have to be strict with yourself to make this happen.

	Person A	Person B
6am		
7	Check SM	Check SM/ Email/Phone
8		
9	Work Starts	Work Starts
10		
11	Check SM/ Email/Phone	
12pm		
1	Check SM/ Email/Phone	
2		
3	Check SM/ Email/Phone	
4		
5	Check SM/ Email/Phone	Check SM/ Email/Phone
6	Work Ends	Work Ends
7	Check SM/ Email/Phone	
8	Watch TV	
9	Watch TV	
10pm	Bed	Bed
	Information overload	Not on information overload
	Constantly distracted	Less distracted

Friends:

If certain people distract you from pursuing your goals, you must quickly stop associating with these people. They're poison and they will be toxic to your sense of motivation. Get rid of your *negative, unimaginative, unambitious, hedonistic, disorganized friends.*

They have a weak mentality because they are slaves to their instincts—they suffer from a pathological need for constant pleasure, instant gratification, and mindless entertainment. They're the type of people who will quickly throw away their dreams if any sort of risk is associated with them. They won't commit to any goals that go against social norms or stand in the way of the next cool party or club event. These people are weak and afraid of their own shadow. Erase their numbers and erase them from your life, immediately.

Instead, you need to find people who are rich in character and education, intensely dedicated and driven, and out to bring change to the world.

Naturally, you should also stay away from the general party/club/bar crowd as well as the more obviously destructive and self-destructive types: drug addicts, people with serious emotional problems, and so on.

Virtuous cycly of activities:

Everything you do in your day must benefit and get you closer to your desire of attaining a perfect body. Avoid activities which will not benefit the pursuit of your desired goal. Doing so will only waste your time and detract from your efforts.

For instance, reading a book on psychology and motivation gets you closer to attaining your desired goal, while reading a fantasy book does not. Why? Because learning about motivation helps you understand how to not get burned out in the pursuit of your desire. Reading a fantasy book, on the other hand, has no relevance to your goals and doesn't get you a step closer to attaining it. Fantasy fiction offers no knowledge that you can apply to get closer to your goal. In fact, reading a fantasy book sets you back, because now you have spent 20 hours or more reading a book, but you are no closer to your goal than before.

This general rule works with everything. Because time is limited, and you want your desire to be fulfilled as fast as possible, everything you do must support your desired goal.

As an example, this is what I did in college:

I wanted to be intellectually accomplished, but I also wanted to be physically fit. Mastering one of those things takes a lifetime, but mastering both takes some serious time management skills, a mature character, and solid planning. You only have 24 hours in a day. You only have one brain, two legs, and two arms.

How could I merge the two without sacrificing either? Well, I thought to myself, I'll pick up the study of psychology. Psychology will teach me about the human mind and how to improve my motivation and confidence. I will become wiser and more educated through the study of psychology, and I will use my knowledge of motivation and confidence to achieve any goal, such as being physically fit and earning straight As.

The sense of wellbeing that results from being physically fit will enhance the quality of all aspects of my life and will thus improve my studies. My improved studies will then enhance my judgment, which will then lead to more intelligent choices and better workouts. Do you see the cycle?

Relationships - should i have them?

In order to live the disciplined lifestyle needed to attain a perfect body and accomplish anything extraordinary, you must stay out of unproductive relationships. If you've had an issue with relation-ships in the past, I would definitely check out **www.journeysofwisdom.com.** The amount of knowledge and wisdom you'll receive there from a single weekend course will far exceed anything you will learn in an over priced college.

I'll break this up into two topics:

Relationships: it's no secret that romantic relationships entail a huge time commitment. In many cases, this is time which could be more productively spent on business ventures, making more money, living an adventurous lifestyle, or in the case of this book – attaining a perfect body.

Let's say we have two equally driven computer scientists that both want to make it to the top of the company. One is in a serious relationship, the other isn't. The single guy has a massive advantage over the one who is in a relationship and here is why: imagine both subjects work equal hours. Once the workday is over, the one in a relationship has to go home and presumably spend a few of the nights with his partner—sharing meals, going to a movie, etc., if he wants the relationship to continue. All this means that he's wasting about 3-4 hours a day doing something that is not going to advance his promotion at work or his career in any way.

On the other hand, the single computer science guy can spend his free 3–4 hours studying new ways of programming, figuring out how to get promoted, and advancing his education by researching and reading in his field. This increases his competency level and eventually leads him to become a master of computer programming. He soon begins to be perceived as the most competent employee in the company. Because of this, he becomes extremely valuable and difficult to replace. He continues his hard work and eventually becomes president of the company—as long as he doesn't get burned out. That's a whole separate topic, though.

What has the guy in a relationship been up to? Well, he got to spend a lot of time with his girlfriend, who later became his wife. He didn't have much spare time to begin with, but after they had their first kid, he definitely had no time at all anymore. He did get promoted here and there, because he is pretty smart, but he's a few levels below the president of the company. It's not really his fault. The relationship took up too much time and he just didn't have as much time and energy to invest into the company as the other guy. He let a few advancement opportunities pass him by because of his family situation, and this also really held him back. Five years later, he ended up divorcing the woman he thought he would love for the rest of his life. Because the relationship is now gone, so is his valuable time investment of 5 years. He basically wasted half a decade and has no progress, professionally, to show for it.

Unless your partner is 100% aligned with your core values and accepts you for who you are and what you're trying to do or be, be warned. Failure in that relationship, long-term, is inevitable. Be patient. Know yourself well.

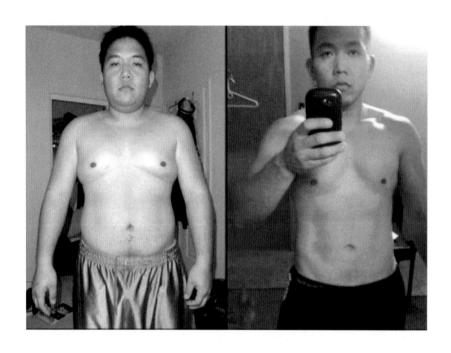

BRANDON LEE

NUTRITION
PROGRAM

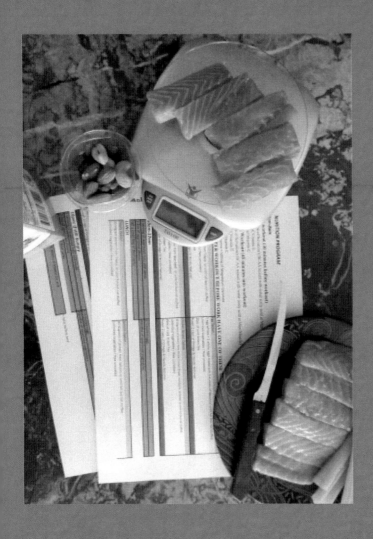

3

Most people find fat loss a mystery. It's not! Really--there isn't that much to it. Here, in the easiest manner possible, I've listed the variables which need to be included in your approach if you want to reduce body fat.

1. Depleting glycogen levels

Glycogen is found in your muscles, as well as in the liver (albeit in very small amounts). When glycogen stores are full, anything you eat will be converted into fat. When glycogen stores are empty, your body will draw upon anything you eat to fill those empty glycogen stores. However, when glycogen stores stay empty for prolonged periods of time, the body then has to tap into its own fat to fill those stores. Thus, if fat loss is your goal, it's advantageous to keep your glycogen levels low, so your body is constantly extracting its own fat to fill those empty glycogen stores.

2. How to deplete glycogen through nutrition

Glycogen is quickly depleted through a low carbohydrate diet, especially one in which the body is completely deprived of sugar (soda, candy, fruit juice, etc.). For the most part, the only thing that replenishes Glycogen are carbohydrates. Sugar, a simple carbohydrate, replenishes glycogen stores the fastest, so to deplete glycogen, I tell my clients that it's extremely important to keep their sugar intake at low levels.

3. What are carbohydrates?

Carbohydrates are divided into two forms: complex carbs and simple carbs. Complex carbs increase your glycogen, but not as fast. On the other hand, simple carbs increase your glycogen very quickly.

Here is a list of complex carbs (somewhat of a threat to fat loss): wild rice, brown rice, steel cut oats, etc.

Here is a list of simple carbs (major obstacles to fat loss): Candy bars, snack cakes, granola bars, hard candy, fudge, chocolate, cookies, bread sticks, crackers, biscuits, soda, sports drinks, most energy drinks, and fruit juice.

4. What's the deal with sugar?

Sugar is by far the number 1 enemy when it comes to fat gain. Sugar is what's making America fat, because it spikes your insulin levels through the roof--more than any other thing you could possibly eat. Keeping sugar at low levels should truly be your number 1 priority if you're seeking to develop a lean and ripped body.

Sugar intake is deceptive. You must become aware of what contains sugar and what doesn't, and be very diligent about reading labels. Once again, if you do not control your sugar intake and keep your sugar intake low, *you will not get ripped.*

Sugar also has other undesirable effects. It ages the skin, decreases energy levels, makes you want more of it after you've consumed some (i.e. sugar is a sugar stimulant), suppresses levels of growth hormone, ages the brain... and of course, as stated above, it causes an increase in body fat.

In short, sugar is bad news and should be avoided.

So how about all the vitamins and minerals you are supposed to get from fruit?

You can easily get all those vitamins and minerals from the abundance of vegetables you'll be eating. In addition, vegetables produce no insulin spike at all, which helps fat loss. This is because, once again, the best way to decrease insulin is to avoid consuming sugar and limiting your overall intake of complex carbs in general.

5. Maintaining a slight caloric deficit

These are the only three things you have to understand about calories.

One: If you're in a state of caloric deficit, you'll always lose weight. If you're constantly losing weight, you are in caloric deficit. You're burning more calories than you're taking in.

Two: If you're in a state of caloric surplus, you'll always gain weight. If you're steadily gaining weight, you are in constant caloric surplus. You're taking in more calories than you're burning.

Three: if you're in caloric maintenance, your weight will remain the same. You're eating just enough so that you will neither lose nor gain weight.

How do I determine how many calories I need to lose weight? Easy, I do this:

Step 1: Take your body weight first thing in the morning on an empty stomach. This is "X". Let's say X is 200 lbs.

Step 2: Take X and multiply by 10, which gives us "Z". In our example, we would multiple 200 lbs by 10, which would give us the number 2,000.

Step 3: Now we take Z and multiply it by 1.1 to get "W". For example, we would take the 2,000 we got above and multiply by 1.1 to get 2,200.

Step 4: Then we take W and subtract 500 to get "Y". Y is the number of calories I would have a general population client eating daily to lose weight consistently. So I would take 2,200 and subtract 500 to get 1,700. 1,700 is the number of calories the client should consume at the beginning.

6. Avoid caloric fluctuations

It's important to avoid dramatic calorie fluctuations in order to keep your metabolism high. You should strive to eat the same quantities of foods consistently. Eating a lot one day and then nothing the next confuses your metabolism, which makes your system more inclined to retain body fat. Also, what's important for fat loss isn't so much what type of calories you eat on a daily basis, but rather your weekly caloric average. That average number is what's really important. For example, you can be spot-on with you diet Monday through Friday, but eat way too much at the weekend, which would actually place your caloric average in a surplus, instead of in the deficit you need to achieve proper fat loss.

Using the example above, let's say you need to eat 1,700 calories daily to lose weight. Let's say you ate 1,700 calories, exactly, Monday through Friday, but ate 2,200 calories on Saturday and 1,900 on Sunday. Your weekly average for that week would be 1,800 calories. It's close to 1,700, but it's not 1,700. So basically you will lose no weight for that week, although you were extremely on point Monday through Friday.

7. Factory-farmed vs organic food

Now that you know how to calculate your calories, it's also important to know how to source your calories. The nutritional profile of factory-farmed food is always going to be worse than organic, especially in its micronutrient profile. On top of that, factory-farmed food exposes you to trace amounts of a myriad of synthetic pesticides, herbicides, fungicides, and insecticides on a daily basis—on top of genetically modified organisms, antibiotics, sex hormones, beta-agonists—and the list goes on and on and on. Instead of factory-farmed food, opt for wild-caught fish, 100% grass-fed beef, and pasture-raised eggs, chicken and turkey. Try to also strive for organic fruits and vegetables—and watch out as well for gimmicky phrases like "cage-free" and "free-range". These mean nothing and just indicate factory-farming operations. You want pasture-raised and organic. To get a more in-depth understanding of how to transition from factory-farmed food to organic, and hopefully one day biodynamic, check out my second book, "Anti-Factory Farm Shopping Guide", which can be found on Amazon or my website **www. trufkinathletics.com**. The book comes with a bunch of instructional videos to give you a more comprehensive understanding of the subject matter.

8. Eat many meals?

In reality, you don't have to eat 5-6 meals per day to optimize fat loss. This is a myth that has been debunked a while back. Hitting your caloric average, what we mentioned above, is what's important and what will determine fat loss. How you distribute those calories doesn't really matter. I try to strive to eat 3-4 meals per day, and that works just fine for me and has for pretty much all of my clients.

9. Low variation in foods

In the beginning, try not to vary your food groups too often because this will make keeping track of your calories very difficult. As you progress and gain more mastery in things like measuring your food, counting your calories, etc., then I would highly recommend that you widen your food groups and change it up as much as possible. If you eat the same food groups constantly for prolonged periods of time, you'll most likely develop gut issues sometime down the line.

10. The fiber factor

The more raw vegetables you eat, the faster you lose weight, the better your skin looks. the longer you live… and so on. Vegetables provide tons of health benefits. One of their key virtues is the tremendous amount of fiber they contain.

The more vegetables you eat, the faster you lose weight and the lower your body fat will be. You cannot gain weight off eating vegetables. Also, when vegetables are eaten at the same time as carbs and fats, the carbs and fats are stored as fat to a lesser extent than when they are eaten without the vegetables.

Because vegetables a lot of fiber, they also act as a great appetite suppressant. In other words, you won't feel hungry as long as you eat plenty of vegetables throughout the day.

Once again, vegetables are extremely important in your fat loss journey, so make sure not to neglect them.

11. The supplement factor

Certain supplements are very useful and should be included in any fat-loss program. It's impossible for me to recommend ideal supplements for any individual reading this book, because I never met that person. So I will just provide a list of supplements I've personally used and have found to work well for me.

WARNING: Consult with a licensed medical professional before taking any of the supplements listed below. These are the supplements I have personally used for myself. The supplements you should be using may differ.

Fish Omega-3	• Dosage: I generally take 5–15 grams a day. • Good brand to buy: Nordic Naturals sells the best Omega-3s on the market. Poliquin Group is also great.
Magnesium Glycinate	• Dosage: I take anywhere between 300 mg and 500 mg daily right 3 times per day. • Good brand to buy: Poliquin Group is awesome.
Vitamin D3	• Dosage: 5,000–10,000 IU per day • Good brand to buy: Poliquin Group
Zinc	• Dosage: 30 mg per day • Good brand to buy: Poliquin Group
Vitamin D3	• Dosage: 5,000–10,000 IU per day • Good brand to buy: Poliquin Group
Whey Protein Isolate	• Dosage: varies widely • Good brand to buy: Poliquin Group
Vitamin D3	• Dosage: 5,000–10,000 IU per day • Good brand to buy: Poliquin Group
ATP Alpha Prime	• Dosage: I take 2 capsules at night. • Good brand to buy: ATP Science
ATP MulitFood	• Dosage: 1 cap per day • Good brand to buy: ATP Science

For quality supplements, the processing methods are more important than whether the supplement is organic or not. So I look for brands that are cGMP and GMP-certified, and if they're also organic that's a huge plus. To know more about how I select supplements and what I look for, check out my second book, "Anti-Factory Farm Shopping Guide".

Fat loss plan

Exact nutritional advice through a book is really tough to give, simply because I never get to meet the reader. It's therefore important to understand that these are plans I've used with my clients or myself, which I've put through detailed assessments before beginning the program. So before carrying out anything you read here, consult with a licensed medical professional. Having said that, here is something that tends to work well for my general population clients:

Step 1: I start my clients off with Plan A for the first 4 weeks. 4 weeks is more than enough, but if the client has 30, 40, or even 50 lbs. or more to lose, I would have the client stay on Plan A for 8–12 weeks. This has worked wonders for a large number of my general population clients.

Step 2: After 4 weeks on Plan A, I would transition the client into Plan B and keep them there for the remaining 12-week program.

To enhance your learning, this book comes with free video instruction. Please email me a receipt of your purchase at **etrufkin@gmail.com** After I receive a picture of your receipt, you will be provided access to the video content.

WARNING: Consult with a licensed medical professional before proceeding with this nutrition program.

NUTRITION PROGRAM

Plan A

First and foremost, I need to find out how many calories the client needs. This is fairly easy to do, but highly dependent on their activity level and the type of work they do. So a guy who works at construction and works out 5 days a week needs way more calories than a computer programmer who doesn't work out at all and sits all day.

So, let's say I determined that one of my 200 lb clients needs 1,700 calories a day to lose weight consistently. The next step would be to determine how to choose the right ratio of proteins, carbs, and fats for those 1,700 calories. For this phase, I would do the following to attain those ratios:

Protein: I take the client's weight in kilograms and multiply by 1.2 grams to get the amount of protein they need daily. In this case, the client would be advised to eat 240 grams daily.

Fat: In this phase, 40% of the calories should come via healthy fats. In this case, that would be 75 grams of fat daily. 1,700 x 0.40 = 680. 680 divided by 9 equals 75.

Carbs: In this phase, I have the client consume zero carbs. However, I would advise the client to eat as many vegetables as they like, hopefully consuming at least 5–6 cups of vegetables daily—ideally organic to reduce their exposure to pesticides. Once again, there's no limit on the carbs.

WARNING: Consult with a licensed medical professional before proceeding with this nutrition program.

Plan B

For plan B, if the client has been consistent with their workouts, and has shown more intensity during their workouts, I simply start adding in the carbs. In our example, I would increase the calories from 1,700 to about 2,100 calories daily and add an extra workout per week. The difference in calories would come from carbs. There are 4 calories in a single gram of carbs—so now the client is doing 5 workouts instead of 4. This person would now be eating 2,100 calories with the following ratio of proteins, fats, and carbs:

Protein: 240 grams/day
Fat: 75 grams/day
Carbs: 100 grams/day

I would have the client have their carbs post-workout, even if the workout was at night. I would still continue to encourage the client to consume a lot of vegetables daily.

QUICK REMINDER

I start a client with Plan A for the first 4 weeks. Four weeks is more than enough, but if the client has 30, 40, or even 50lbs or more to lose, I have them stay on the Plan A for 8–12 weeks.

ROUGH EXAMPLE OF A TYPICAL NUTRITION LAYOUT FOR

Plan A

7am: Meal 1
3 whole eggs (pasture-raised, organic)
1 avocado (organic)
10am: Meal 2
1 scoop of Whey Protein Isolate (Poliquin)
1pm: Meal 3
16 oz of chicken breast (pasture-raised, organic)
2–3 cups of vegetables of choice
4pm: Meal 4
1 scoop of Whey Protein Isolate (Poliquin)
7pm: Meal 5:
10–12 oz of sockeye salmon
2–3 cups of vegetables (organic)
3 liters of artesian water

Plan B

7am: Meal 1
3 whole eggs (pasture-raised, organic)
1 cup of steel-cut oats (Organic)
1 avocado (organic)
10am: Meal 2
1 scoop of Whey Protein Isolate (Poliquin)
1pm: Meal 3
16 oz of chicken breast (pasture-raised, organic)
2–3 cups of vegetables of choice
4pm: Meals 4
1 scoop of Whey Protein Isolate (Poliquin)
7pm: Meal 5:
10–12 oz of sockeye salmon
2–3 cups of vegetables (organic)
3 liters of artesian water

Note

If you're not used to eating vegetables, I would recommend cooking or boiling them lightly before consuming them. Cutting them up into small pieces may also really help.

Another important thing to remember is you have to factor your cooking oils into your total calories. For example, one tablespoon of extra virgin olive oil could contain as much as 120 calories.

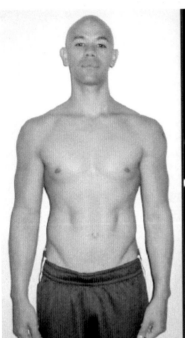
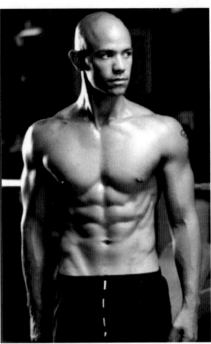

ZAI HOLDER

WORKOUT
PROGRAM

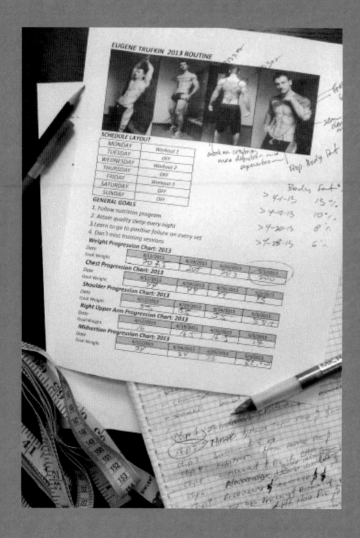

4

Just like with a proper nutrition program, it impossible to provide a general program that suits everyone's needs. A workout programs needs to be specifically tailored to the individual and their capabilities and limitations. However, there are some general rules that anyone can follow to enhance their fat loss and not waste too much time figuring it all out.

1. You have to deplete glycogen levels:

Glycogen is found in your muscles but is also present in your liver in very small amounts. When glycogen stores are full, anything you eat will be converted into fat. When glycogen stores are empty, anything you eat will be diverted to fill them instead of body fat. Also, when glycogen stores are empty, your body extracts its own fat to fill those stores. The process of extracting stored body fat to fill empty glycogen stores is a key variable in losing fat.

So what's the most effective workout for depleting glycogen/burning fat?

Least Effective
Aerobics
Excessive cardio
Yoga

Moderately Effective
Cardio that isn't done to excessive levels
Calisthenics

Most Effective
Weight training
Sprinting

As you can see, weight training and sprinting are most effective at burning fat. To be more specific, the weight training routine should be structured in the following manner:

Short rest intervals

For best fat loss results, rest intervals between sets should be between 60 seconds and 120 seconds.

Large compound movements

For best fat loss results, mainly incorporate compound movements such as the barbell deadlift, squat, bench press, leg press, etc. Stay away from focusing too much time on small muscle groups such as the biceps. You'll burn more glycogen by incorporating compound movements.

High volume for best results: The more sets you incorporate into your routine, the more fat you will burn—generally speaking. Great sleep, nutrition, and low stress levels should be taken into consideration for this to really work though.

Reps: For best fat loss results, the ideal repetition range should be 8 to 12. In general, avoid focusing exclusively on very low repetition ranges (1–4 reps), and very high repetition ranges (25 and above).

Weight training has the following advantages that all other forms of exercise simply cannot provide.

Growth Hormone

Weight training increases the amount of growth hormone in your body. This hormone is responsible for burning fat--the more growth hormone you have, the faster you burn fat.

Testosterone

Weight training also increases the amount of testosterone in your body. Testosterone is responsible for building muscle and boosting sex drive. The more testosterone you have, the more muscle you will be able to obtain, with less effort. The less testosterone you have, the less muscle you will be able to build.

Staying Anabolic

Weight training can be very anabolic, when incorporated in conjunction with great sleep and nutrition. It's a different story with cardio and aerobic exercise, which both have the potential to burn muscle and thus decrease your metabolism, and therefore make fat gain that much easier. In other words, weight training builds muscle mass and makes you leaner; cardio and aerobics break it down and can make you fatter.

Magazine Cover Looks:

I'm guessing everyone reading this book wants to look, to some degree, like the guys on the cover of fitness magazines. They want rock hard muscle, six-pack abs, and superlative definition and muscle separation. Let's face it--you're definitely not going to achieve that by doing excessive cardio and aerobics. To achieve that look, you have to lift weights. There are no ifs or buts about it. If you don't lift weights, you're not going to look muscular and ripped.

Defying Genetics:

The good thing about weight training is that it allows anyone to transform the way their body looks. In a sense, it allows them to reprogram their genetically determined shape. If you have narrow shoulders because of a narrow bone structure, you can make them wider by weight training your shoulders and back muscles, building a wider frame. You can extend this transformation to every part of your body, and the only way to do that is through weight training. Cardio, yoga and aerobics will not do that.

Work Around Injuries:

Weight training allows you to work around injuries. For instance, if you have lower back pain, simply avoid exercises that activate the lower back—until that lower back is properly corrected. On the other hand, cardio and aerobics make it very difficult, if not impossible, to spare specific body areas and work around your injuries.

Having said all the above, once again, it's important to note that it's impossible to create an individualized training program for anyone reading this book, simply because I don't know exactly who's reading this. So the best I can do is outline a 12-week workout plan that I've found generally successfully with a large portion of my clients.

THE FAT LOSS WORKOUT PROGRAM IS DIVIDED INTO 3 PLANS:

Plan A
Plan B
Plan C

Each of the plans lasts 4 weeks. I would start my client on plan A and then progress to plan C. If the client hasn't reached their goal by the end of plan C (client has 50 or more pounds to lose) then I would have them return to plan A and progress through the plans again until the desired body fat level is reached. I would change the exercises slightly and concentrate on improving training focus and intensity. I would constantly emphasis that the most important aspect of a training program is actually the nutrition—not the training. No caloric deficit = no fat loss.

Once you've reached your desired body fat level and general body composition, it's time to really bring out the full aesthetic potential of your body. The following will explain how to go about doing so.

1 Take a look at your body in the mirror and honestly evaluate your entire physique. Ideally, you want to take pictures from as many angles as possible as well. Figure out what you want to work on the most and what will really enhance the aesthetic appeal of your body. Remember, aesthetics is all about balance. If you feel that your chest is overdeveloped compared to the rest of your body, you probably don't want to work on your chest as much. If that is the case, you probably want to work more on your shoulders and back instead, to create a more balanced appearance.

2 For best results, you want to concentrate on enhancing one muscle group at a time. If you try to enhance too many muscle groups at once, the results you experience will not be as rapid as they would be if you concentrated on the development of one muscle group at a time. So if you want to improve your chest, concentrate on improving that area for 12 weeks, and then if you feel like it's developed to the degree you want it to be, move on to another muscle group and maintain your chest from there on.

3 Once you've finished enhancing one muscle group, reevaluate your body and select a new muscle group to work on. Repeat this process indefinitely.

WARNING: Consult with a licensed medical professional before proceeding with this nutrition program.

WORKOUT PROGRAM: PLAN A

PLAN A: BEGINNER

Notes

I really try to emphasize to my clients that cardio isn't necessary to lose fat. If your nutrition and diet are on point, there is really no reason to do heavy amounts of cardio. At most, I have my clients doing 15–20 minutes of cardio before every workout. Most of my clients I have doing no car-dio at all. Remember, proper nutrition and hitting that caloric deficit are key. A lifestyle that facilitates your health and wellness goals helps attaining that caloric deficit and eating properly that much easier. Also, you must keep reminding yourself that fat gain is a symptom of poor lifestyle and nutritional choices. Approach fat loss at the root cause to have lasting change. Anything outside of that will only produce short-term results. Long term, you will always relapse.

I would have my clients follow this phase for 4 weeks, typically working out only 4 times a week. I try to have my clients focusing heavily on proper nutrition, sleep, and general rest and recovery. Most people these days are in a state of constant chronic fatigue, and the last thing you want to do is throw them into a high volume routine and deplete the very little energy they have left.

To enhance your learning, this book comes with free video instruction. Please email me a receipt of your purchase at **etrufkin@gmail.com** After I receive a picture of your receipt, you will be provided access to the video content.

General weekly layout
Monday: Workout 1
Tuesday: Workout 2
Wednesday: OFF
Thursday: Workout 3
Friday: Workout 4
Saturday/Sunday: OFF

Workout 1 - Upper	Week 1	Week 2	Week 3	Week 4 Deload
A1: Overhead Barbell Press	5 sets of 8-10 reps	5 sets of 8-10 reps	5 sets of 8-10 reps	5 sets of 8-10 reps
rest 120 seconds				
B1 Bent Over Barbell Rows Supinated	5 sets of 8-10 reps	5 sets of 8-10 reps	5 sets of 8-10 reps	5 sets of 8-10 reps
rest 120 seconds				
C1 Flat Dumbbell Chest Press	4 sets of 10-12 reps	4 sets of 10-12 reps	4 sets of 10-12 reps	4 sets of 10-12 reps
rest 90 seconds				
C2 Single Arm Dumbbell Rows	4 sets of 10-12 reps	4 sets of 10-12 reps	4 sets of 10-12 reps	4 sets of 10-12 reps
rest 90 seconds				
D1 Flat Bench EZ Bar Tricep Extensions	3 sets of 10-12 reps	3 sets of 10-12 reps	3 sets of 10-12 reps	3 sets of 10-12 reps
rest 60 seconds				
D2 Standing EZ Bar Bicep Curls	3 sets of 10-12 reps	3 sets of 10-12 reps	3 sets of 10-12 reps	3 sets of 10-12 reps
rest 60 seconds				
Workout 2 - Lower	Week 1	Week 2	Week 3	Week 4 Deload
A1 Barbell Reverse Lunges	5 sets of 8-10 reps	5 sets of 8-10 reps	5 sets of 8-10 reps	5 sets of 8-10 reps
rest 120 seconds				
B1 Barbell Hip Thrust	4 sets of 10-12 reps	4 sets of 10-12 reps	4 sets of 10-12 reps	4 sets of 10-12 reps
rest 90 seconds				
C1 Lying Leg Curls	4 sets of 8-10 reps	4 sets of 8-10 reps	4 sets of 8-10 reps	4 sets of 8-10 reps
rest 60 seconds				
D1 Seated Calf Raises	3 sets of 12-15 reps	3 sets of 12-15 reps	3 sets of 12-15 reps	3 sets of 12-15 reps
rest 60 seconds				
E1 Half Kneeling Cable Rotations (low to high)	3 sets of 10-12 reps	3 sets of 10-12 reps	3 sets of 10-12 reps	3 sets of 10-12 reps
rest 60 seconds				
Workout 3 - Upper	Week 1	Week 2	Week 3	Week 4 Deload
A1: Bench Press	5 sets of 8-10 reps	5 sets of 8-10 reps	5 sets of 8-10 reps	5 sets of 8-10 reps
rest 120 seconds				
B1 Bent Over Barbell Rows - Pronated	5 sets of 8-10 reps	5 sets of 8-10 reps	5 sets of 8-10 reps	5 sets of 8-10 reps
rest 120 seconds				
C1 60 degree Incline Dumbbell Press Pronated	4 sets of 10-12 reps	4 sets of 10-12 reps	4 sets of 10-12 reps	4 sets of 10-12 reps
rest 90 seconds				
C2 Single Arm Dumbbell Row	4 sets of 10-12 reps	4 sets of 10-12 reps	4 sets of 10-12 reps	4 sets of 10-12 reps
rest 90 seconds				
D1 External Dumbbell Rotations	3 sets of 10-12 reps	3 sets of 10-12 reps	3 sets of 10-12 reps	3 sets of 10-12 reps
rest 30 seconds				
Workout 4 - Lower	Week 1	Week 2	Week 3	Week 4 Deload
A1 Leg Press High/Narrow Stance	5 sets of 8-10 reps	5 sets of 8-10 reps	5 sets of 8-10 reps	5 sets of 8-10 reps
rest 120 seconds				
B1 Barbell Hip Thrust	4 sets of 10-12 reps	4 sets of 10-12 reps	4 sets of 10-12 reps	4 sets of 10-12 reps
rest 90 seconds				
C1 Standing Calve Raises	4 sets of 10-12 reps	4 sets of 10-12 reps	4 sets of 10-12 reps	4 sets of 10-12 reps
rest 60 seconds				
D1 Half Kneeling Cable Rotations (middle)	3 sets of 12-15 reps	3 sets of 12-15 reps	3 sets of 12-15 reps	3 sets of 12-15 reps
rest 0 seconds				
D2 Stability Ball Crunch	3 sets of 10-12 reps	3 sets of 10-12 reps	3 sets of 10-12 reps	3 sets of 10-12 reps
rest 60 seconds				

WORKOUT PROGRAM: PLAN B

PLAN B: INTERMEDIATE

Notes:
The volume in this routine is a bit higher than in the previous one. For this reason, at this point I tell my clients it's important to really enhance the quality and consistency of sleep and focus heavily on proper nutrition, especially nailing down that slight caloric deficit. Workouts in and of themselves will produce no results unless sleeping and nutrition are on point. You cannot train out a bad lifestyle. Having said that, this routine is 4 weeks long and should be a progression of the previous routine.

To enhance your learning, this book comes with free video instruction. Please email me a receipt of your purchase at **etrufkin@gmail.com** After I receive a picture of your receipt, you will be provided access to the video content.

General weekly layout
Monday: Workout 1
Tuesday: Workout 2
Wednesday: OFF
Thursday: Workout 3
Friday: Workout 4
Saturday: Workout 5
Sunday: OFF

Workout 1 - Upper	Week 1	Week 2	Week 3	Week 4 Deload
A1: Incline Bench Press	5 sets of 6-8 reps	5 sets of 6-8 reps	5 sets of 6-8 reps	5 sets of 6-8 reps
rest 120 seconds				
B1 Bent Over Barbell Rows Pronated	5 sets of 6-8 reps	5 sets of 6-8 reps	5 sets of 6-8 reps	5 sets of 6-8 reps
rest 120 seconds				
C1 Flat Dumbbell Chest Press	4 sets of 8-10 reps	4 sets of 8-10 reps	4 sets of 8-10 reps	4 sets of 8-10 reps
rest 90 seconds				
C2 Single Arm Dumbbell Rows	4 sets of 8-10 reps	4 sets of 8-10 reps	4 sets of 8-10 reps	4 sets of 8-10 reps
rest 90 seconds				
D1 15' Incline Dumbbell Fly- Pronated	3 sets of 8-10 reps	3 sets of 8-10 reps	3 sets of 8-10 reps	3 sets of 8-10 reps
rest 60 seconds				
D2 Seated Face Pull - Rope	3 sets of 8-10 reps	3 sets of 8-10 reps	3 sets of 8-10 reps	3 sets of 8-10 reps
rest 60 seconds				
Workout 2 - Lower	**Week 1**	**Week 2**	**Week 3**	**Week 4 Deload**
A1 Barbell Reverse Lunges	5 sets of 6-8 reps	5 sets of 6-8 reps	5 sets of 6-8 reps	5 sets of 6-8 reps
rest 180 seconds				
B1 Leg Press High/Sumo Stance	4 sets of 12-15 reps	4 sets of 12-15 reps	4 sets of 12-15 reps	4 sets of 12-15 reps
rest 90 seconds				
C1 Lying Leg Curls	4 sets of 6-8 reps	4 sets of 6-8 reps	4 sets of 6-8 reps	4 sets of 6-8 reps
rest 60 seconds				
D1 Leg Extensions	4 sets of 10-12 reps	4 sets of 10-12 reps	4 sets of 10-12 reps	4 sets of 10-12 reps
rest 60 seconds				
E1 Seated Calf Raise	4 sets of 15-20 reps	4 sets of 15-20 reps	4 sets of 15-20 reps	4 sets of 15-20 reps
rest 60 seconds				
F1 Ab Roller	4 sets of 10-12reps	4 sets of 15-20 reps	4 sets of 15-20 reps	4 sets of 15-20 reps
rest 60 seconds				
Workout 3 - Upper	**Week 1**	**Week 2**	**Week 3**	**Week 4 Deload**
A1: Bench Press	5 sets of 6-8 reps	5 sets of 6-8 reps	5 sets of 6-8 reps	5 sets of 6-8 reps
rest 90 seconds				
A2 Standing Curls with Ez Bar Supinated	5 sets of 6-8 reps	5 sets of 6-8 reps	5 sets of 6-8 reps	5 sets of 6-8 reps
rest 90 seconds				
B1 Close Grip Bench Press Smith Machine	4 sets of 8-10 reps	4 sets of 8-10 reps	4 sets of 8-10 reps	4 sets of 8-10 reps
rest 90 seconds				
B2 Standing Dumbbell Curls Supinated	4 sets of 8-10 reps	4 sets of 8-10 reps	4 sets of 8-10 reps	4 sets of 8-10 reps
rest 90 seconds				
C1 Cable Tricep Pushdown EZ Bar	3 sets of 10-12 reps	3 sets of 10-12 reps	3 sets of 10-12 reps	3 sets of 10-12 reps
rest 60 seconds				
C2 Cable Bicep Curls with EZ Bar	3 sets of 10-12 reps	3 sets of 10-12 reps	3 sets of 10-12 reps	3 sets of 10-12 reps
rest 60 seconds				

Workout 4 - Lower	Week 1	Week 2	Week 3	Week 4 Deload
A1 Leg Press High/Narrow Stance	5 sets of 6-8 reps	5 sets of 6-8 reps	5 sets of 6-8 reps	5 sets of 6-8 reps
rest 120 seconds				
B1 Lying Leg Curls	4 sets of 6-8 reps	4 sets of 6-8 reps	4 sets of 6-8 reps	4 sets of 6-8 reps
rest 90 seconds				
C1 45' Back Extenions	4 sets of 12-15 reps	4 sets of 12-15 reps	4 sets of 12-15 reps	4 sets of 12-15 reps
rest 90 seconds				
D1 Standing Calf Raise	4 sets of 10-12 reps	4 sets of 10-12 reps	4 sets of 10-12 reps	4 sets of 10-12 reps
rest 60 seconds				
E1 Leg Raises	3 sets of 10-12reps	3 sets of 10-12reps	3 sets of 10-12reps	3 sets of 10-12reps
rest 0 seconds				
E2 Situps	3 sets of 10-12reps	3 sets of 10-12reps	3 sets of 10-12reps	3 sets of 10-12reps
rest 60 seconds				
Workout 5 - Upper	Week 1	Week 2	Week 3	Week 4 Deload
A1: Incline Chest Press Machine	4 sets of 8-10 reps	4 sets of 8-10 reps	4 sets of 8-10 reps	4 sets of 8-10 reps
rest 60 seconds				
B1 Dips	4 sets of 8-10 reps	4 sets of 8-10 reps	4 sets of 8-10 reps	4 sets of 8-10 reps
rest 60 seconds				
C1 Hex Press	3 sets of 8-10 reps	3 sets of 8-10 reps	3 sets of 8-10 reps	3 sets of 8-10 reps
rest 10 seconds				
C2 Dumbbell Fly - Pronated	3 sets of 8-10 reps	3 sets of 8-10 reps	3 sets of 8-10 reps	3 sets of 8-10 reps
rest 90 seconds				
D1 Seated Dumbbell Laterals	4 sets of 30 reps	4 sets of 30 reps	4 sets of 30 reps	4 sets of 30 reps
rest 0 seconds				
D2 Cable Face Pull	4 sets of 8-10 reps	4 sets of 8-10 reps	4 sets of 8-10 reps	4 sets of 8-10 reps
rest 90 seconds				

WORKOUT PROGRAM: PLAN C

PLAN C: ADVANCED

Notes:

This is a progression of Plan B. Once again, even at this point, I make sure to focus heavily on educating my clients that the most important aspects of a training routine are lifestyle and nutrition. Working out only really works when those two things are in place. I make sure their sleeping is on point (sleeping between the hours of 10pm and 6am), they're diligent with keeping track of their calories, they're well hydrated, and they have good time-management skills. This program is going to be 4 weeks long.

To enhance your learning, this book comes with free video instruction. Please email me a receipt of your purchase at **etrufkin@gmail.com** After I receive a picture of your receipt, you will be provided access to the video content.

General weekly layout
Monday: Workout 1
Tuesday: Workout 2
Wednesday: OFF
Thursday: Workout 3
Friday: Workout 4
Saturday: Workout 5
Sunday: OFF

Workout 1 - Upper	Week 1	Week 2	Week 3	Week 4 Deload
A1: Bench Press	6 sets of 6,6,4,4,2,2	6 sets of 6,6,4,4,2,2	6 sets of 6,6,4,4,2,2	6 sets of 6,6,4,4,2,2
rest 120 seconds				
B1 Bent Over Barbell Rows - Supinated	6 sets of 6,6,4,4,2,2	6 sets of 6,6,4,4,2,2	6 sets of 6,6,4,4,2,2	6 sets of 6,6,4,4,2,2
rest 120 seconds				
C1 Seated Dumbbell Shoulder Press	4 sets of 4-6 reps	4 sets of 4-6 reps	4 sets of 4-6 reps	4 sets of 4-6 reps
rest 90 seconds				
C2 Single Arm Dumbbell Row	4 sets of 4-6 reps	4 sets of 4-6 reps	4 sets of 4-6 reps	4 sets of 4-6 reps
rest 90 seconds				
D1 Lying Tricep Extensions - Ez Bar	3 sets of 6-8 reps	3 sets of 6-8 reps	3 sets of 6-8 reps	3 sets of 6-8 reps
rest 60 seconds				
D2 Standing Barbell Curls - EZ Bar	3 sets of 6-8 reps	3 sets of 6-8 reps	3 sets of 6-8 reps	3 sets of 6-8 reps
rest 60 seconds				
Workout 2 - Lower	Week 1	Week 2	Week 3	Week 4 Deload
A1 Barbell Reverse Lunges elevated	6 sets of 4-6 reps	6 sets of 4-6 reps	6 sets of 4-6 reps	6 sets of 4-6 reps
rest 120 seconds				
B1 Barbell Hip Thrust	4 sets of 4-6 reps	4 sets of 4-6 reps	4 sets of 4-6 reps	4 sets of 4-6 reps
rest 90 seconds				
C1 Lying Leg Curls	4 sets of 4-6 reps	4 sets of 4-6 reps	4 sets of 4-6 reps	4 sets of 4-6 reps
rest 90 seconds				
D1 Seated Calf Raise	3 sets of 8-10 reps	3 sets of 8-10 reps	3 sets of 8-10 reps	3 sets of 8-10 reps
rest 60 seconds				
E1 Stability Ball Lower Leg Raise	3 sets of 12-15 reps	3 sets of 12-15 reps	3 sets of 12-15 reps	3 sets of 12-15 reps
rest 10 seconds				
E2 Stability Ball Crunch	3 sets of 10-12 reps	3 sets of 10-12 reps	3 sets of 10-12 reps	3 sets of 10-12 reps
rest 60 seconds				
Workout 3 - Upper	Week 1	Week 2	Week 3	Week 4 Deload
A1: Bench Press	6 sets of 6,6,4,4,2,2	6 sets of 6,6,4,4,2,2	6 sets of 6,6,4,4,2,2	6 sets of 6,6,4,4,2,2
rest 120 seconds				
B1 Bent Over Barbell Rows - Pronated	6 sets of 6,6,4,4,2,2	6 sets of 6,6,4,4,2,2	6 sets of 6,6,4,4,2,2	6 sets of 6,6,4,4,2,2
rest 120 seconds				
C1 30' Incline Dumbbell Press	4 sets of 4-6 reps	4 sets of 4-6 reps	4 sets of 4-6 reps	4 sets of 4-6 reps
rest 90 seconds				
C2 30' Incline Dumbbell Rows Neutral	4 sets of 4-6 reps	4 sets of 4-6 reps	4 sets of 4-6 reps	4 sets of 4-6 reps
rest 90 seconds				
D1 Dumbbell Lateral Raise	3 sets of 6-8 reps	3 sets of 6-8 reps	3 sets of 6-8 reps	3 sets of 6-8 reps
rest 60 seconds				
D2 30' Incline Prone Lateral Raise	3 sets of 6-8 reps	3 sets of 6-8 reps	3 sets of 6-8 reps	3 sets of 6-8 reps
rest 60 seconds				

Workout 4 - Lower	Week 1	Week 2	Week 3	Week 4 Deload
A1 Leg Press High/Narrow Stance	6 sets of 6,6,4,4,2,2	6 sets of 6,6,4,4,2,2	6 sets of 6,6,4,4,2,2	6 sets of 6,6,4,4,2,2
rest 120 seconds				
B1 Barbell Hip Thrusts	4 sets of 6-8 reps	4 sets of 6-8 reps	4 sets of 6-8 reps	4 sets of 6-8 reps
rest 90 seconds				
C1 Standing Calf Raise	3 sets of 6-8 reps	3 sets of 6-8 reps	3 sets of 6-8 reps	3 sets of 6-8 reps
rest 60 seconds				
D1 Squat / Low to High Cable Rotation	3 sets of 8-10 reps	3 sets of 8-10 reps	3 sets of 8-10 reps	3 sets of 8-10 reps
rest 10 seconds				
D2 Stability Ball Crunch	3 sets of 8-10 reps	3 sets of 8-10 reps	3 sets of 8-10 reps	3 sets of 8-10 reps
rest 60 seconds				
Workout 5 - Upper	Week 1	Week 2	Week 3	Week 4 Deload
A1: 60' Incline DB Fly - Pronated	4 sets of 8 reps	4 sets of 8 reps	4 sets of 8 reps	4 sets of 8 reps
rest 60 seconds				
B1 Olympic Barbell Preacher Curls	4 sets of 6,6,4,4 reps	4 sets of 6,6,4,4 reps	4 sets of 6,6,4,4 reps	4 sets of 6,6,4,4 reps
rest 10 seconds				
B2 Overhead EZ Barbell Tricep Extensions	4 sets of 10 reps	4 sets of 10 reps	4 sets of 10 reps	4 sets of 10 reps
rest 120 seconds				
C1 Seated Face Pulls - rope	3 sets of 10 reps	3 sets of 10 reps	3 sets of 10 reps	3 sets of 10 reps
rest 60 seconds				

QUICK REMINDER

Sometimes one of my clients needs to lose 40 or more pounds. The more body fat the client needs to lose, the longer it will take them to lose it. I usually try to never have clients lose more than 2 pounds a week. So, if the client has finished plan C and still needs to lose more weight, one thing I might do is simply have them repeat plan a through plan C once more. The second time around though, I would up the intensity and the weights on every exercise.

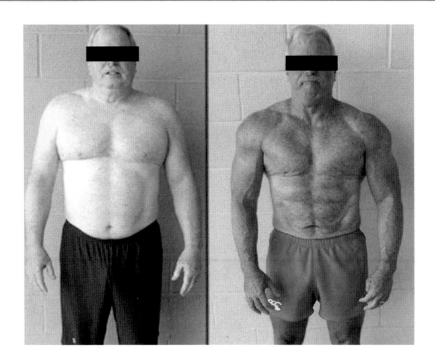

JOHN WALSH

MAXIMIZE THE PROGRAM

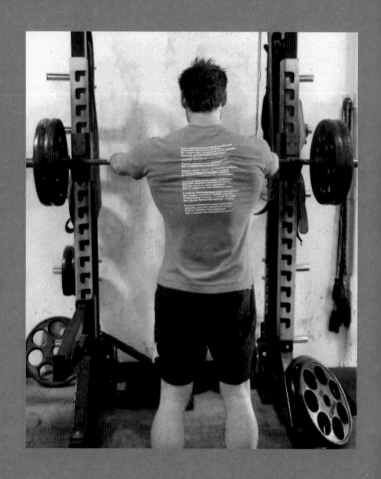

5

Mind-muscle connection:

This is by far one of this program's most important aspects to master. If there is one secret that a person with a great physique can share, it is the mind-muscle connection. Some people "get it" right from the start, and others take a while to understand it. The mind-muscle connection is basically the ability to feel a specific exercise working a muscle that you intend to work. Basically, if you don't feel the muscle (the one you are intending to grow or improve) being worked it will not grow or improve. It's as simple as that.

These are the steps you need to take to develop a mind-muscle connection.
To simplify the process, let us concentrate on the barbell biceps curl:

Step 1: Google "barbell biceps curl anatomy" and look at pictures of which muscle groups are being used, and how they're used. This will give you a good understanding of the exact muscle groups this exercise is supposed to target. (Learning about anatomy in further detail is great, but not necessary. You just need to know the basics.)

Step 2: Set up your exercises in front of a mirror. While performing the bicep curls, look at the muscle in the mirror the entire time.

Step 3: Start performing the bicep curls and really concentrate on how the barbell and its motion are affecting the biceps, the muscles you intend to grow.

Step 4: During the motion, don't rely on the barbell for resistance. Rather, deliberately squeeze the bicep as hard as you can throughout the entire range of motion. In other words, squeeze the bicep all the way up and all the way down. Don't just throw the weight on the way down.

Step 5: Continuously flex the bicep throughout the entire set, without a break in the flexion. While flexing, really hone in mentally on the biceps. Your mind should be focused on nothing but your biceps-- everything else should be invisible to you at this point. The only thing you should be perceiving mentally and physically is your bicep. Make sure to be present to the sensation inside the muscle and really feel each individual muscle fiber flexing.

Step 6: In order to really feel each rep in the muscle, each one should last 5 seconds and the entire set should be at least 21 seconds of continuous flexion. Flexion below the 21 second threshold produces less muscle development.

Step 7: After the set is finished, put down the barbell, and flex the bicep in the mirror from many different angles.

Step 8: Repeat this technique for all other muscle groups.

These steps must be taken to master the mind-muscle connection. Use every training session to practice this technique, in order to master it eventually. You need to master the mind-muscle connection in order to succeed.

Master the basics:

When people see someone who has an admirable physique, they may presume it's because that person uses "special" exercise(s) to achieve that look. That presumption couldn't be further from the truth. You have to understand that it's not the type of exercises you do that makes a difference; what's important is how you do those exercises. Learning how to really maximize basic lifts (deadlifts, squats, bench press, overhead press, etc.) is far more important and far more productive than learning how to use a buso ball, do some kind of silly one-legged stance while overhead pressing, or anything along those lines. My advice is to really master the basic lifts and forget about everything else.

Here are some illustrations of the importance of mastery vs. lack of mastery.

Example of a person who HAS NOT mastered the barbell bench press:

This person doesn't have a well thought-out routine for the bench press. He basically just arrives at the gym and then decides he wants to bench that day. He does 12 reps on the bench-- he could easily do 20, but stops at 12, thinking that will be enough. He simply goes through the motions and has no mind-muscle connection. He doesn't feel it in his chest, and he has no understanding of how the bench press could develop his body. In between sets, he checks out other people, watches TV, checks Facebook on his phone, daydreams about the next party or thinks about a work project. This person will see no results and is completely wasting his time.

Example of a person who HAS mastered the barbell bench press:

This person shows up to the gym with a game plan for the bench press. In fact, he already thought out his entire bench press routine days beforehand. He has a predetermined number of reps, sets, and rest times between sets. He even knows how fast he's going to do reps. He has a solid understanding of how the bench press works the chest, shoulders, and triceps.

He understands that if he positions his elbows at a certain angle, he'll feel the movement more in the chest muscles than he would if he positioned his elbows differently. Since he wants to target the chest, he knows exactly which angle to use. When he does the bench press, his mind is 100% focused on targeting the right muscle groups and really making them burn in order to get a solid pump. In between sets, he concentrates on nothing but the next set. He is 100% absorbed in the workout and doesn't pay attention to anything outside of it. This person will see magnificent results and obtain a well developed chest. He is making optimal use of his time, and he has definitely mastered the exercise.

INTENSITY:

Intense muscular contractions are the single most important variable in charge of getting muscles to grow fast. You really have to know how to take yourself over the top and conquer intensely painful workouts in order to have an insanely developed physique. Weak workouts will give you weak results. Extreme workouts will give you extreme results. It's a pretty simple concept that most people refuse to truly acknowledge.

How can I attain these "intense muscular contractions"?

I could easily write an entire book on intensity, its importance and benefits, and what intensity really means. However, to keep it simple, I'm just going to describe it in one small phrase: positive failure. I want you to make sure to attain positive failure on most sets you do during the workouts.

What's "positive failure"?

There are two portions to any lift that you should be concerned with: the positive portion and the negative portion. On a pressing exercise, such as a shoulder dumbbell press, the positive motion is when you're pressing the weight up and the negative motion is when you're bringing the weight back down.

On a pulling motion, such as a lat pull down machine, the positive is when you're pulling the weight down and the negative is when you're bringing the weight back up.

Your goal is to always achieve positive failure. Going all the way to positive failure will produce enough intensity for your body to make rapid changes. Not reaching positive failure will produce mediocre results at best, or possibly even no results.

These are some common indicators that your intensity ISN'T great enough:
1. You're able to carry on a conversation between sets. This is the biggest indicator. If you're doing it right and going to positive failure, you'll most likely be out of breath.
2. Finishing a set and feeling like you could have easily done 4-5 more reps during that set.
3. You end the exercise when it becomes too difficult.
4. You end the set because a chosen number of reps have been completed, but you have not yet reached positive failure.
5. Your workouts last two or three hours and you're able to train 6-7 days a week. You can't work out hard and long. Either your workouts are long, or your workouts are hard... It will be one or the other. If you're really pushing hard, 45 minutes to an hour is more than enough per workout, with 4-5 workouts per week, maximum. The less time you spend in the gym to get the desired result, the better.

How do you know if your intensity is up to standard?
Don't just strive to do your best, because your best might not be good enough. Rather, strive to do what's humanly possible. Consult YouTube videos of guys like David Goggins, Doug Miller, Arnold Schwarzenegger, Branch Warren or Johnnie Jackson. Their workouts, mindset, and intensity are 100%-- this is exactly how you need to be to achieve the best results. On a scale of 1 to 10, they're all at level 10, all of the time. That's why they're champions and legendary figures in their sport. If you're not up to par with these guys, you must figure out a way to close the gap and emulate their behavior and intensity patterns as closely as possible for best results. The further you are from their level of intensity, the less likely you will be to experience any admirable results. If you're in the 8-10 category, you're good to go. If you're below an 8, you need to figure out a way to progres-sively up your intensity.

Reminder:
Intensity should be understood as more than just the physical effort you expend at the gym. The definition of intensity, in my opinion, also encompasses the amount of focus you are able to muster in the gym. What are you doing in between sets? Are you checking your text messages, or visualizing yourself performing the next set with extreme, brutal energy? What are you doing during the set? Are you just going through the motions and trying to get the reps out of the way, or are you really focusing on every single inch of the movement, every single rep, and how each rep is affecting your targeted muscle group? Are you in the gym today to just get this workout out of the way, or are you in the gym today to get one of the best workouts in of your life?

Here are some ways to increase your intensity:
The Card Trick, Again!
This is a powerful, easily implemented tool that can help direct your thoughts and keep you focused on your goal. Use note cards to write down the following reminders, and read them before entering the gym. The glove compartment of your car is a convenient place to leave these cards.

Write the following on a card, and read it before entering the gym:

Upon entering the gym, I will not make eye contact with anyone. I will be 100% focused on the workout ahead of me, and how I can maximize that workout.

I will remember to bring my workout program with me, and already know ahead of time what needs to be done during that workout.

I will make sure to attain positive failure on every single set during the workout.

I will use my rest periods, between sets, to focus on my next set.

I will make sure to establish the mind-muscle connection on every set.

I will leave my phone in the car, so I am not bothered during my workout.

I will not talk to anyone during the workout.

Ritualize your Workouts:

Create a motivational video montage for yourself:

This is another excellent, easy technique that can be used to increase your intensity in the gym. Find a cool video that really gets you pumped every time you watch it. This video should be like a short trailer of sorts--no more than 3-5 minutes long. You can find millions of these on YouTube or Vimeo.

For the longest time, I really liked watching "The Best of Kevin Levrone" on YouTube right before my workouts. The video content and music really got me fired up, and I noticed a tremendous increase in my intensity level and overall enthusiasm and energy in the gym. It made me feel like a monster!

Find a training partner who is more intense and dedicated than you:

Finding a person who is way more badass and hardcore than you are is another great way of increasing your intensity--and on top of that, it will increase your accountability. Don't select someone who is a chatterbox. Also, this person should preferably have more knowledge than you as well.

You don't need to train with this person every day; it may be difficult to match up schedules consistently, and because of that it can become more of a headache than an aid. Ideally, you should aim to train with this person once or twice a week, and train on your own the rest of the time.

Use Great Music:

Listening to inspiring, energizing music is another way to amplify your intensity levels to the max and beyond.

Change Up Your Environment:

Changing up your workouts is important, but changing up your training environment is equally important, although it doesn't need to be done nearly as frequently as varying workouts.

Most people are on a tight schedule, and changing stuff up, even to a minor extent, always throws off your time efficiency until you adapt to the new schedule and environment. These are the layouts and strategies I have found to work best.

Option 1: Have three different gym locations that you cycle through. Stick with each location for a month and rotate to a new location at the beginning of a new month.

Option 2: Stick with the same gym, but once every two weeks or so, do one training session in at a different gym--preferably one which has a completely different training environment and appearance.

Option 3: Buy a pair of adjustable dumbbells and fit in an outdoor workout from time to time. It doesn't have to be done consistently--just enough to break up the pattern of things and spark your motivation and enthusiasm for training. I typically pick a close friend or two and turn the training session into an all-day event. We pack up the dumbbells into a car and all drive down to a nearby forest or beach. We bring plenty of food and drinks with us as well. For a couple of hours we enjoy running around the wilderness, doing workouts with the dumbbells, and just generally having a great time while being physically active.

I love the connection I feel with the wilderness. It feels so natural, and it always allows me to reconnect with my basic human instincts. Once the sun starts to go down, we throw a barbecue with the food we brought with us and enjoy nature in the cold night temperatures as well. I would usually only do this once every 2-3 months, but it is always extremely fun, and always works to remotivate me for another month or two of training in an indoor gym.

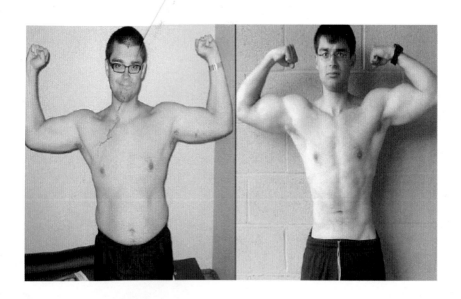

DMITRI ARKHIPOV

REJUVENATION

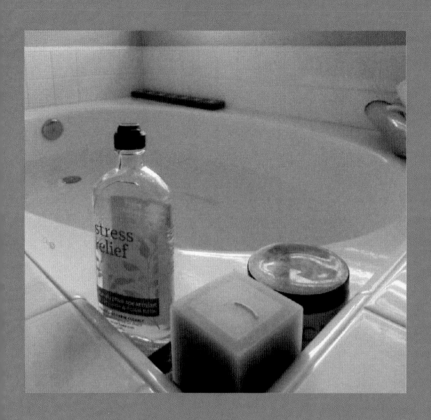

6

To get the most out of a training routine, you need to be able to properly recover from your workouts and keep your body well-rested through the weeks and months of intense workouts. Remember, the more intense your workouts, the more seriously you need to take your recovery. Sleeping well is a great start, but if you really want to be able to recover fully, I would recommend the following measures.

Massages:

I'm a great believer in having at least one or two massages per month. Ideally, if you have the funds, try to have one every week or two. If you train hard, your body is always going to be extremely tight and tense. Muscles that are tight for prolonged periods of time are always subject to injury. A quality massage is a great way to overcome this tightness.

Art therapy:

ART Therapy (Active Release Therapy) is becoming more popular and widely used. If a muscle is put through an intense workout session, it shortens and becomes very tense, and does not allow blood to flow effectively through the muscle tissue. When blood doesn't flow easily through muscle tissue, toxins aren't filtered out and the muscle isn't allowed to properly recover. ART Therapy is meant to elongate the overly trained muscle tissue, increase blood flow into the targeted muscle, and thus restore the muscle to a healthy state. I would highly recommend ART Therapy. It is also covered by most health insurance programs.

Hot baths:

Hot baths are very important. Not only do they help your body feel rejuvenated and increase blood flow, reducing the amount of toxins in the body, but if taken at night before bed, they also help you get a great night's sleep. Try to take at least one 45-minute hot bath per week, ideally on a Sunday night before bed. That way, when the week does begin, you feel rejuvenated and well rested. Hot baths also lower your cortisol levels, and make your skin look younger and healthier.

Here are some ways you can set up your bath to optimize relaxation and recovery benefits:
1. What you need: candle lanterns, a few cheap candles, Epsom bath salts, a bathtub, and a drink made up of 2 liters of cold water flavored with 1 lemon, and a few raspberries.
2. Place candles in the lanterns and position as desired around the bathtub.
3. Fill up the bath with relatively hot water and pour in Epsom salts.
4. Position your 2 liter drink near the tub so it's readily accessible to you.
5. Light the candles in the lanterns, turn off electric lights, and close all the doors.
6. Soak in the water for 45 minutes, trying not to think about anything. Just relax and clear your mind.

Sun exposure and vitamin D3

Moderate sun exposure is great at relaxing you and reducing stress, and can be very rejuvenating as well. The sun is a natural source of vitamin D3, a vitamin responsible for various immune functions as well as better, healthier looking skin. Don't fear; sun exposure for short periods of time is actually healthy for you. It strengthens the functioning of your immune system and boosts your overall energy. Sun exposure for prolonged periods of time, on the other hand, is extremely damaging and can have an aging effect on your skin.

My recommendation is to try to have one 20–30 minute sunning session per week. Don't use sunscreen and make sure to cover your face with a thick towel or shirt. Try to get your exposure from the sun, not from tanning beds. Once again, just like with the baths, try to enjoy a peaceful moment while lying in the sun. Use it as a mini-nap in the middle of the day, if you can. Don't attend to your phone or other activities during this time. What's more, you don't have to be directly in the sun. Just finding shade under a tree will also provide you with great sun exposure and minimize the risk of sunburn.

Sleep

It's always tough to address sleeping problems because there are several different kinds of sleep pathologies. Some people have trouble falling asleep, some people have trouble staying asleep, and some people sleep for 6, 8, or even 10 hours and still do not feel rested. Although scientists don't yet know everything there is to know about the exact benefits of sleep to the human body, one thing is for certain: If you don't sleep well you're going to be miserable and your body will also age faster. Generally, your body repairs itself physically from the hours of 10:30pm to 2am, and it repairs itself mentally from the hours of 2am to 6am. Because of this, it's important to try to sleep between the hours of 10:30pm and 6am very consistently. This is very, very important. If your sleeping patterns are terrible, your life will be miserable. Worse still, you will never be able to recover fully between workouts no matter how good your eating is. If you want to know more about the importance of sleep, check out Joe Rogan's podcast with Matthew Walker. It'll be life-changing—I promise. Matthew Walker's book, "Why We Sleep: Unlocking the Power of Sleep and Dreams" is also amazing.

How to Achieve Perfect Sleep

The importance of letting your body wake up naturally at least one day a week

People tend to force their bodies to wake up when the body is not ready to awaken and go to bed when it's not ready to sleep. In other words, they're not working with their body's natural sleeping cycle. One way to break the artificial, fatigue-inducing cycle and feel more rejuvenated is to simply allow your body to wake up whenever it feels like waking up at least once a week. In other words, just don't set the alarm clock.

The importance of getting a short midday nap at least once a week

If you can afford to, and you feel a little tired, just let your body doze off during the middle of the day for 20-25 minutes, once or twice a week. By letting your body rest whenever you feel tired, you help keep up the natural energy cycle and thus optimize your body's health and well-being. If you do this, you will also look less haggard. Drinking coffee when you're in a state of fatigue will only make you look more haggard and accelerate aging.

Sleep, Anxiety, and Stress

Anxiety and stress have severe effects on sleeping patterns. 99% of sleep disorders are due to varying degrees of anxiety and stress. If you're suffering from poor sleep, I guarantee that you're most likely suffering from some degree of anxiety or stress. This is a really tricky subject to address, but my best advice is that you work very proactively at curing your anxiety and stress. Do not presume that it's going to go away on its own. Try to understand that anxiety is a symptom of some type of root cause. Try to approach the problem at the root, instead of constantly being in a symptom-management mindset. An example of a symptom-management mindset would be someone who takes anxiety medication but continues to work a job that causes their stress and anxiety to shoot through the roof. This approach would only worsen the symptoms as time went on because the problem was never solved at the root cause. If this is a serious issue for you, check out the following resources:

John McMullin at *www.journeysofwisdom.com*
Jator Pierre at *www.wehlc.com*

The fallacy of work hard/play hard, and why that idea leads to quicker aging, low energy, fat gain, and burnout

You often hear the phrase, "Work hard, play hard." The next time someone says that to you, take a good look at that person's appearance and general health and well-being. Most likely, for lack of a better phrase, they look like crap. They look many years older than they actually are. They're often haggard and worn out, their skin looks like they've had a recent bout with the black plague, and a good 90% of those who use the phrase "Work hard, play hard" are overweight. The reason for their poor physical condition is that they work really hard, long, stressful hours during the week and fail to sleep enough all week because of those stressful work hours—then when the weekend rolls around, they get even less sleep, drink even more, and eat even more unhealthily.

Having a direction and extreme purpose in life

Nothing works better at easing the mind and improving sleep and overall quality of life than having some kind of goal to strive for intensely—a goal that really means something to you, and that you really want to attain. When this goal is established, you will notice that your direction in life will become clear and your daily actions will take on more meaning. Once this happens, you will notice that your mind is more at ease, and you will have an easier time going to sleep. Once you dedicate your body and mind to something, you are likely to perceive life as more meaningful and less complicated. Just remember, you can be worth billions—but if you have no meaning in your life, you will always be miserable. If what you're doing has no meaning to YOU, it's a complete waste of time 100% of the time. If you really think about what I just said, you will not be able to deny that simple fact.

Attending to Basic Biological Needs

The human body evolved to function in a nomadic lifestyle, constantly roaming the earth, hunting, pursuing adventure and facing danger, and eating a seasonal diet of variable wild-caught foods. In other words, humans need to be physically active and mentally stimulated through novel experiences. If they aren't, an accumulation of frustrated energy will form, leading to anxiety, which can later surface as depression. Depression can cause some people to oversleep, but for others, depression and anxiety can cause insomnia. If you suffer from insomnia, maybe a lack of adventure and physical activity is the root cause of your sleeping disorder. Get your body into better alignment with its natural drives and instincts, and many anxiety symptoms will sort themselves out. At the end of the day though, find out what's causing your anxiety at the root. Stay away from symptom-management strategies.

The Ideal Sleeping Environment

You want your brain to associate your room with a peaceful, restful environment. If your brain associates your room with entertainment and wakefulness, you'll have a harder time falling asleep. Here is my advice: don't keep a TV or use any other entertainment devices in your room. Make sure your room is completely dark and noise free when you go to bed. The less your mind associates your room with wakefulness and the more it associates it with sleep, the better. Try to use very dim Edison lights, instead of the harsh and overly bright lights typically available.

Stimulants and Sugar and Their Effects on Energy and Sleep:

Energy drinks or other caffeinated beverages can affect the quality of your sleep, even if they are taken early in the morning. Everyone's central nervous system is different and sensitivity levels differ as well. Carryover effects can occur too. If you are sensitive to caffeine, the energy drink you have on Monday can still be interfering with your sleep on Tuesday.

Other Tips To Help You Sleep Better:

Don't watch violent films before bed or do anything that is likely to cause a spike in adrenaline.

Don't do work that stresses you out or makes you nervous before bed time.

If you need 8 hours of sleep to feel rested, go to sleep 8 and a half hours before your scheduled waking time. This will allow you 30 minutes to fall asleep.

Try to do something relaxing for the last hour or two before bedtime. Clear your mind. I love reading books and listening to podcasts before bed. I love the Joe Rogan Podcast, Podcasts with Paul Chek, and my podcast Art of Strength and Mind.

Another aspect to consider is you want to lay motionless in bed and try to just concentrate on your breathing, relaxing your muscles. Try not to fidget, move around or think about anything outside of your breathing and physical relaxation. Usually, if you start tossing and turning and moving around in bed, you'll be less likely to fall asleep.

Ideal sleeping pattern

Ideally you want to go to sleep and wake up at the same time every day. You don't want your sleeping patterns to be sporadic - this is a surefire way to prevent sleep from fulfilling its restorative purpose.

Supplement yourself to sleep:

I personally avoid using any sleep medication. Poor sleep has a cause, and 99% of time it's a form of continuous worrying which leads to anxiety and stress. You want to find the root of the problem and solve it at that level. Remember, try to avoid symptom management strategies. They provide short term symptom relief at the expense of long term success and health.

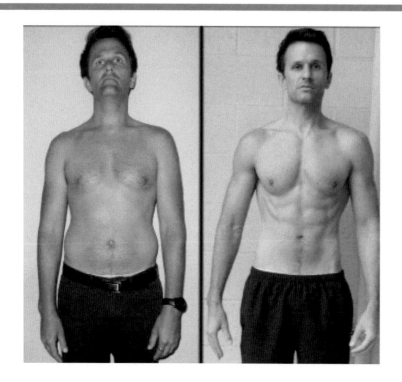

KEVIN CONROY

STRESS
AND FAT
GAIN

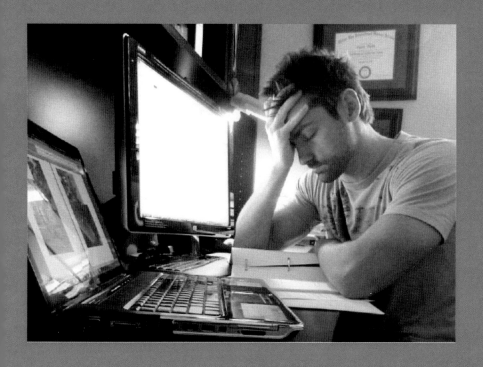

7

Stress and its effect on your body and appearance

Hormones play a major role in determining how you look. High levels of testosterone will give you a square jaw, larger muscles, and more body hair. High estrogen levels will give you soft facial features and little body hair. High levels of a stress hormone called cortisol can also transform the way you look. Cortisol is a hormone released into your body when you're mentally stressed. In high amounts, it will damage your physical appearance as well as your wellbeing.

High cortisol levels can do the following to your body:
1. Make your skin look older
2. Give you wrinkles, pimples, rashes, dark circles and bags under your eyes
3. Contribute to hair loss
4. Lower sex drive and reduce overall energy throughout the day
5. Make it impossible for you to attain quality sleep
6. Cortisol can further transform your body's appearance. Instead of distributing fat equally over the entire body (as it would be otherwise), your body will tend to store fat only around the mid-section. This will give your body an apple shape.

More problems caused by cortisol:
1. Even with the aid of the best trainer, fat loss becomes nearly impossible. The fat just never seems to come off.
2. Cortisol decreases muscle mass, thus making your body appear less toned. You will look softer and weaker.
3. Also important, but not as imminent if you are young: high cortisol levels dramatically increase your chances of a stroke or heart attack. They can also cause immune suppression (you get sick very frequently and easily), ulcers, cancer, and uncontrollable, consistent headaches and muscle tension.
4. Cortisol decreases testosterone (the masculinity hormone), decreases sex drive, decreases growth hormone, which is responsible for muscle repair and fat loss, and increases depression and anxiety.

There are TWO important facts to consider when trying to understand how mental stress affects you and how cortisol can negatively affect your appearance.

One, the Central Nervous System (CNS), which is responsible for regulating stress, can't tell the difference between physical stress (running away from a serial killer) and mental stress (dealing with a hostile or unprofessional boss). It responds to all stressors in exactly the same way: by releasing a massive amount of cortisol into your body.

Two, the CNS has a slow recovery process. Your CNS doesn't handle repeated stressors very well if it isn't given a few weeks to months to recover between stressors. It hasn't evolved to do this. Instead, your CNS has evolved for this pattern:
•   You're chased by a huge mountain lion for a few minutes.
•   You escape the mountain lion.
•   Nothing too upsetting happens for a few months.
•   Repeat.

The above structure is a totally healthy pattern for your body—one that your nervous system can easily regulate. The key variable is that it must have enough time to recover from stressful episodes. Instead, however, this is what typically happens in today's environment:

At the beginning of the month, you spend several days feeling stressed out about finishing work projects on time. Your CNS is taxed. It reacts by dumping a huge amount of cortisol in your body.

By the middle of the month, you're still stressed out about finishing projects on time and your CNS has not recovered. Then something goes badly wrong with your workplace software system, which causes you to lose a lot of the work you recently completed and sets you back quite a bit. Your CNS is taxed again! More cortisol is released, adding to the already large amount of cortisol coursing through your body.

At the end of the month, workplace tensions boil over and you have some serious conflicts with your coworkers. Your CNS is taxed even more, and it wasn't even given enough time to recover from the stress accumulating since the beginning of the month. You realize another month has gone by and you haven't done anything enjoyable; the only thing you've done is work (a synopsis of the last couple of years of your life). This thought makes you feel terrible and causes you to question your life choices, so your CNS is taxed again, still without being given time to recover from the previous stressors. Now there is a massive amount of cortisol in your body around the clock.

Having to pay your mortgage causes you even more stress.

Your company starts restructuring. You fear you may be on the list for the next round of layoffs. Although you don't enjoy your job, you still need that paycheck to pay the bills. You tell yourself you're screwed if you keep this job, and screwed if you don't. More cortisol is released. You were overburdened before, but now you're in Armageddon mode.

You get the picture. And that's just one month. Add a couple of years to that pattern and you'll be looking really messed up. I haven't even included the stresses involved in parenting, relationships, or the countless things that can go wrong in life--car problems and other unexpected expenses, injury, death of a loved one, etc. Just the things listed above are more than enough to deplete your body's ability to regulate stress and cause an excess of cortisol in your body at all times.

What you need to take away from this

The CNS has not evolved to be able to sustain the long, long hours of low-control, high-pressure office work typically seen in today's corporate environment, especially in middle-management type positions. This is one of the leading reasons burnout is so prevalent in today's corporate environment. Burnout refers to a person hating their job and/or losing interest in it, having chronic fatigue, etc. Long hours, lack of meaningful work, lack of balance in life because work consumes so much time, office politics, not feeling appreciated at work and not enough control or say all contribute to the mess.

75% of people in America are considered overweight. Some people would blame bad nutrition, but cortisol, which is a byproduct of work-related stress, is the real culprit. Cortisol causes you to want starchy and sugary foods. It stimulates those unhealthy cravings. The more cortisol you have in your body, the more you want that crappy food. And the more you consume of that crappy food, the more weight you gain. It's a pretty simple process, really.

Look, I'm not preaching a countercultural way of life. In fact, I support a hardworking, structured, lifestyle. However, science shows that ideally, for optimum health, people should be living a no-madic-type lifestyle filled with physical activity, organic foods, novel experiences, and a balanced range of activities, because this is how humans have evolved to live. Even standing desks in the office force you into static positions. The human body has evolved to be dynamic in its movement—not static.

Science shows that our current life conditions—demanding work environments, jobs that involve sitting all day, fast food diets—are destructive to our health. We simply have not evolved to live this way. Having such an unnatural lifestyle will cause serious health problems.

Just imagine a flower trying to grow through a layer of concrete in order to reach the sunshine at the top. What happens is that the flower is forced to grow out of the cracks in the concrete. Result: the flower grows crooked, mangled, and puny. Office work is the concrete. You are the flower. Don't take my word for it. Just look around you. Step outside anymore in America and you'll see that 9 out of 10 people are full of mental and physical pain—full of disease and obesity. Just look at their faces and you'll see that their souls must have escaped them a long time ago. Lifeless and constantly haggard, they just wonder throughout their days like zombies—one paycheck into the next. And that's the story behind how cortisol works, when it's produced in your body, and why it alters your appearance. Don't listen to me. Hear what the guys with the Ph.Ds have to say and watch the documentary Stress, Portrait of a Killer (2008). It's available on Amazon, or can be watched on YouTube for free.

More key cortisol facts

Cortisol is actually released in response to physical effort as well. However, the amount of cortisol produced this way is a small, negligible fraction of the amount of cortisol produced by mental stress. Long distance running, long duration cardio and aerobics tend to produce the most cortisol in your body (among physical stressors, that is). Don't let a trainer sell you on the idea that working out is a one-stop shop for decreasing stress. This is simply not the case. In fact, many studies show working out can actually increase stress (and therefore cortisol) levels. For instance, if a person who doesn't like to lift weights is forced to lift weights, his or her cortisol level will go through the roof during every training session. The lesson: don't do a certain type of exercise, no matter how beneficial, unless you enjoy that type of exercise. You have to find the type of exercise that suits you best—find something you like. This being said, long distance running (running for more than 30 minutes at a time) seems to increase cortisol levels the most, compared to all other forms of exercise, such as lifting weights.

Finally… It sounds like I'm bashing corporate/office work. In a sense, yes, I am, simply because I've seen corporate America rob so many people of their vitality and youth over and over again. Corporate work seems to have a way of sucking the soul out of people's bodies, even the most motivated. Most people simply have not evolved to function well by spending most of their time sitting behind a desk, working crazy hours and juggling demanding schedules.

Look, I just want people to know their daily existence doesn't have to be that way. Life is SHORT. If a 9 to 5 (more like 7 to 6) office job isn't right for you, then get the heck out. You don't have to do that in order to make a living or to get the things you want. Find an occupation which works for you. You might lose a little money upfront, but at least you'll be true to yourself (something most of us claim to do, but very few actually do).

«We all make choices, but in the end, our choices end up making us»- Andrew Ryan

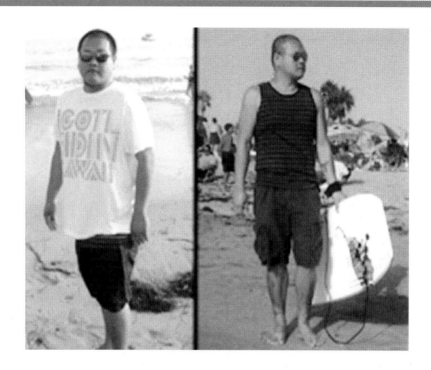

MIKE REYES

FAT LOSS TRICKERY

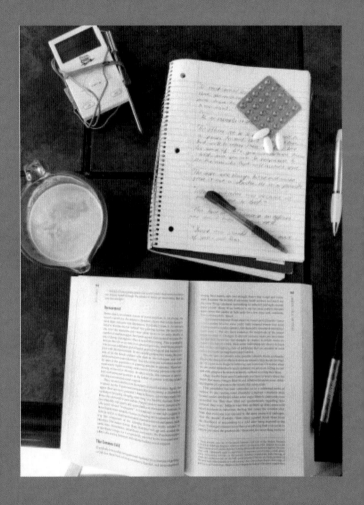

This chapter covers some very effective, but less widely-known ways to shed body fat and achieve a body fat percentage in the ultra-low range. As a side note, everything suggested here should be done under professional supervision.

Fat loss trickery

On occasions, I do have certain clients do a day of fasting here and there. This is done on a case-by-case basis depending on the client's needs and abilities. As mentioned before, since I don't know exactly who's reading this book, it's impossible for me to say whether this is an appropriate strategy for you specifically.

First, I establish a base daily calorie intake and base meal quantity for about 4 weeks. In other words, I advise my client consume the same amount of calories per day and the same number of meals per day, eaten at the same times during the day if possible. Once again, I advise my client to be very consistent about eating the same number of calories every day and the same number of meals every single day for this to work.

Presuming the client is consistent with the instructions above for 4 weeks, on the 5th week I will maintain those similar eating habits Monday through Saturday, but on Sunday the client would con-sume no food. I mean no food whatsoever—a complete fast. I will follow this pattern for about 2 to 3 weeks, with one fasting day per week, and then return to a normal eating schedule. I never do this for longer than 3 weeks.

On Sunday, instead of eating food, I will fill up a gallon container with ice-cold water and mix in the following supplements: 1–2 scoops of BCAAs. Sip on the gallon of ice-cold water throughout the day, making sure to finish it by the end of the day.

Here is an example of what the 5th week should look like:

Monday – 1,500 calories – divided into 6 meals
Tuesday – 1,500 calories – divided into 6 meals
Wednesday – 1,500 calories – divided into 6 meals
Thursday – 1,500 calories – divided into 6 meals
Friday – 1,500 calories – divided into 6 meals
Saturday – 1,500 calories – divided into 6 meals
Sunday – No food, no meals

Side note: Severely cutting your calories for prolonged periods of time compromises your metabolism, making you gain more body fat and lose muscle.

The cold and training in Ukraine

Training in cold temperatures elevates the amount of calories you burn, because the cold causes your body to increase its heat production dramatically to keep your core body temperature up, thus expending more calories. For instance, if you have two people with the exact same body type, but one person works out in a warm climate and the other works out in a cold climate, the one in the cold climate will burn a great deal more calories doing the same exact workout.

I experienced the effects of cold weather on fat loss first hand while living in Ukraine, where temperatures are very cold most of the year, dropping well below zero in winter. During those colder periods, I noticed myself getting more and more shredded despite doing basically the same workouts, following the same nutrition protocol and keeping the same lifestyle patterns. The only changed variable was that the weather was extremely cold, instead of warm or hot.

In short, working out in cold weather could be the answer for those who have trouble losing fat or who are struggling to lose that extra 3-4lbs of unwanted fat around the midsection. This is with the presumption, of course, that you have absolutely everything else nailed down-- such as nutrition, keeping stress levels low and training consistently. If you don't live in a cold climate, you can always try working out in the very early morning, drinking ice water throughout the day, especially first thing in the morning, swimming in a very cold swimming pool, or taking ice baths or very cold showers on a regular basis.

Beyond your normal blood work, here is a list of tests you would generally want done:

Total Testosterone

Free Testosterone

LH (Luteinizing hormone)

FSH (Follicle-stimulating hormone)

Estradiol

SHBG (Sex hormone-binding globulin)

Thyroid and liver function tests and Cortisol test

Tricks I don't recommend: the truth about steroids

Let's be honest. The reason steroids are so popular among bodybuilders is that they work—in their own way.

What steroids cannot do is make you into a hard, disciplined worker, which is what's really going to make you succeed. Nor will they allow you to be intense in the gym.

They also won't improve your gym intelligence, which is probably one of the most important variables that are usually overlooked. They're not a shortcut, because they certainly won't educate you on proper training, nutrition, mental game, and supplementation. In fact, if you start a steroid cycle making stupid workout choices, all you're going to do is grotesquely exaggerate the results of those stupid choices.

My personal advice is to avoid steroids: they're illegal and they're unhealthy. Frankly, what is the point of investing insane amounts of time, money and effort to get a "perfect", i.e. awesomely strong, younger-looking and healthy-looking body by using measures which can hurt your health?

However, steroid use is indisputably the elephant in the room in bodybuilding. I believe the truth is a better basis for good choices than denial or scaremongering, and this is why I'm giving you the straight story here and addressing the most common questions and myths about steroids—in the hope that you will see that the healthy options offered earlier in this chapter are a better choice.

Are steroids safe?

It depends what you mean by "safe."

Will the smallest dose instantly turn you into a raging lunatic, destroy your life and ravage your body? No, of course not. It is definitely possible to limit the undesirable effects of steroids if they are conservatively used, e.g. at lower dosages, infrequently, and for shorter periods of time. However, it is almost inevitable that users will experience some side effects. Serious health problems are most likely to arise if you take steroids in significant dosages for prolonged periods of time, or if you are one of those rare few that have a predisposition to have a negative reaction to any amount of steroids.

The problem is that there is no way to guarantee that you won't be one of the unlucky ones. It can also be harder than you may realize to stay conservative in your usage.

And this is why, once again, I neither use steroids nor endorse their use.

For an extreme example of what large doses of steroids can do to your health, just look at Andreas Munzer. His autopsy photos can be found on Google. Upon his death, at the young age of 31, doctors found collapsed organs, numerous tumorous growths on his liver, and nonexistent testicles. Munzer died a very painful death. If you mess with steroids, they will mess with you.

Do steroids make your penis small?

No. However, steroids do make your testicles appear smaller. During a cycle of steroids, the user's testicles will retract into the body at least to some degree. However, this effect can be reversed and if the user stops taking steroids, the testicles will drop down into their normal position.

I've heard steroids can have negative effects on physical appearance. Is this true?

It depends. If you're genetically predisposed to have hair loss or acne, steroids will only exaggerate those problems. For instance, if you have minor hair loss already, steroids could easily make all of your hair fall out. If having a full head of hair is important to you, this is not a chance you want to take. To be fair, however, steroids aren't known for causing baldness out of the blue in users who didn't have a pre-existing tendency to suffer from hair loss. Similarly, if you suffer from acne naturally, you'll probably see a dramatic increase in breakouts—bigger, more severe breakouts, too. But if you don't have bad skin to begin with, you aren't all that likely to get terrible breakouts on steroids.

Aren't steroids illegal?

That's right. As stated above and as per the Anabolic Steroids Control Act of 1990, steroids are 100% illegal, and if you are caught with them you will face arrest and prosecution. The police will treat you the same way as they would treat a person caught with heroin or cocaine.

Final Word:

Before attempting a cycle, just make sure you have your basics mastered. Your sleeping should be on point, your understanding of nutrition and workout science should also be great, drop that stressful job that's lowering your testosterone, and make sure you're doing it for all the right reasons. Don't be another tool in the gym.

So where do people get them? Is there a black market for steroids?

Some users are able to obtain a prescription from a TRT therapist. (TRT therapists also have a booming trade in treating guys whose steroid abuse has messed up their body to the point that it can no longer produce normal hormones without help—yet another aspect of the potential for trouble in this area.)

Those who aren't able to get a prescription have to resort to obtaining steroids from the black market. This can be tricky, not to mention sometimes dangerous. The main risks are the following:

The market is flooded with counterfeit steroids that look like the real thing, and are labeled and packaged like the real thing, but are not the real thing. They are often just made in someone's basement, and it's anyone's guess what is actually in that vial. If you're lucky, your counterfeit purchase will simply be ineffective. If you're unlucky, you could be facing some serious health consequences.

(B) Because the Anabolic Steroids Control Act of 1990 ended the activities of law-abiding, casual steroid dealers who were simply selling to their gym buddies to fund their own steroid habit, the void instead was mostly filled by guys who were the real deal: full-time, "career" drug dealers. It goes without saying that we are talking about extremely shady characters who only have profit in mind. If you plan to obtain steroids through the black market, you will most likely have to deal with these people at one point or another. They'll smile at you, they'll act like your friend, and they'll say all the right stuff, but don't be fooled – they're shady as can be. They don't give a toss about you or your health—all they're interested in is your money.

So what do steroid users actually do? What do they take?

Users might do a cycle lasting anywhere between 8 and 12 weeks and typically take biweekly injections of steroids such as testosterone enanthate, a slow-acting hormone also given in legitimate medicine to older male patients whose body no longer produces enough testosterone naturally. More experienced users might add a second anabolic steroid.

Those who are able to find a doctor who doesn't disapprove of the practice and is willing to advise them will do this under his or her supervision, and cautious users typically start with the lowest possible dosage. Other, less cautious users may get their information from internet forums or by asking other bodybuilders for pointers. As you can imagine, this approach carries a fairly high level of risk, and it's easy to get bad advice (or misunderstand good advice) with dangerous consequences.

It is also common for steroid users to take other hormones and drugs as part of their bodybuilding program. For instance, hCG (Human Chorionic Gonadotropin) and Arimidex (anastrozole) are often taken off-label as part of the course of treatment to try to enhance muscle growth and definition, and to limit or reverse some of the undesirable effects of the steroids—even though it should be noted that these products have side effects of their own, which can be problematic.

OK, I agree all this sounds like quite the chemistry experiment… But surely all steroid users aren't recklessly mainlining large amounts of the stuff. Isn't there such a thing as conservative use?

Of course. For example, first time users will typically limit their cycle of use to a period of 8 weeks. Conservative users will start with the lowest possible dosages, again in order to manage unpleasant side effects and more serious health risks.

However, a typical beginner, even one using precautions, would still have an extensive (and expensive) shopping list. Here is a fairly standard example of the supplies involved:

- Testosterone Enanthate
- Human Chorionic Gonadotropin, aka hCG
- Arimidex
- 23 gauge needles
- 3ml syringes
- Bacteriostatic water

As you can see, our guy is now taking quite a serious amount of stuff. In fact, he is probably taking more shots and pills than your average 80 year old grandpa. If he is (rightly) concerned about side effects, he'll systematically have a full blood panel done before and after each cycle of steroid use in an effort to avoid adverse health effects or treat them when they occur. *Of course, even this offers no guarantee that the effects can be prevented or reversed; there is no such thing as a completely prudent and foolproof approach to steroids.*

Will taking steroids transform my out-of-shape body?

No. Most "successful" users (the ones who see dramatic results) have trained naturally for a few years with extreme discipline and intensity before even thinking about using steroids. If you've trained for less than 8 years, it's a little stupid to do a cycle. You haven't mastered the foundations to really optimize those drugs anyway.

I'm 19 and healthy as a horse. Surely there's nothing I do now that can have serious long-term effects on my body?

Think again. For one thing, even dedicated steroid users would advise against starting steroids under the age of 25, because your natural testosterone levels continue to progress until that age, and taking artificial steroids can interfere with that progression, reducing your potential.

Moreover, drug reactions are never predictable. It could help to get complete blood work done before and after a cycle, to objectively determine the effects of a drug on your body and try to predict future effects. However, the only real way to know how your body reacts to a certain drug is simply to take that drug.

I've been using steroids for a while and am experiencing some worrying side effects. What should I do?

Stop your usage immediately and seek medical help right away. Don't mess around with steroids because if they are misused (e.g., injected in the wrong spot) or overused, they will mess you up, possibly permanently. Who are you trying to impress anyway? Will those people even remember you a few weeks after you've died? Probably not. Not worth it. Gain some confidence.

I know it's not very healthy, but isn't it just a lot easier to inject some steroids for a while rather than go through this whole process of doing research and educating myself about fitness, nutrition and so on?

Ironically, no, it's not that easy at all. Steroid use requires its own research—it's actually a complicated process. It's not as easy as just taking a pill here or there or injecting something into your ass once a month. Injection points, quantities, type of needle, dosage, timing, and many other factors have to be considered. It's pretty elaborate and requires a lot of in-depth knowledge.

If you're hoping to do this with medical supervision, you will have to go through the delicate process of finding a TRT (Testosterone Replacement Therapist) who can be convinced to help you.

If you're going the black market route, it's going to be tough to buy your products from a reliable and trustworthy source. You can't afford to be fooled by cool personalities just because they're friendly and seem to care about you. They could be an undercover cop, or they could be selling you garbage that will kill or disable you upon injection. You'll have to really do your research and be extremely cautious.

(Not to mention, none of the steroid-related research or knowledge actually helps you learn how to work out, eat properly and sustain motivation, so you'll have to do all that anyway.)

The bottom line

I've been as low as 5-8% body fat without the use of any steroids whatsoever--and so have hundreds and thousands of other people, who have experienced amazing results without even coming close to a vial of steroids.

I was able to achieve amazing results without using any of this stuff, and I honestly believe you can too. Just because you might not have the best genetics doesn't mean you're not going to have that body you've always wanted. All it means is that you have to try harder and work smarter for that dream to come true. If you're lost, hire a coach. I've had many coaches in my life that helped accelerate my learning curve a tremendous amount. If you're going to take the steroid route anyways, do it through a licensed doctor.

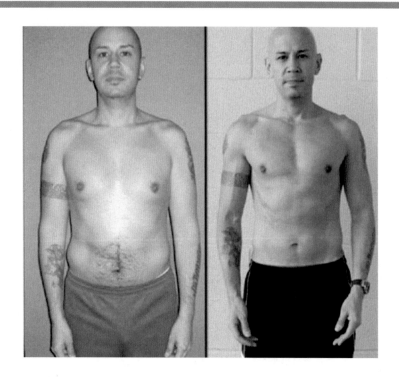

BRIAN BICE

LOOK
LIKE
SUPERMAN

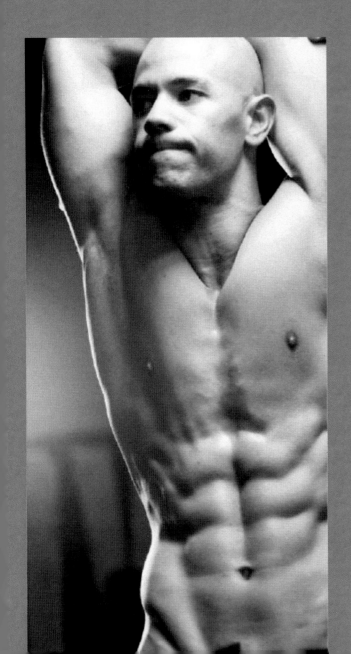

9

Maintaining a low body fat percentage and staying fit offers a tremendous number of health benefits. However, there are many other benefits you will likely experience as a result of being fit—many of which are not so openly discussed.

Attract the attractive

Yes, it's true. We're visual creatures, and a significant part of attraction is due to appearance. By improving your appearance, you'll be able to attract more desirable, attractive partners without changing anything else about yourself. In fact, just by having an aesthetically appealing body you'll have people coming up to you, starting more conversations with you, and just generally showing more interest in you and how you live your life. And since people in our society are becoming ever fatter, unhealthier and more out of shape, with even young people seeing the effects of processed food and unhealthy lifestyles in their complexion, hair, posture and so on, you'll become an even rarer and more sought-after commodity.

Sex is more fun

Another great perk of being fit is that people will actually enjoy having sex with you a lot more. Your partner(s) will generally be really turned on by you.

Be the leader

As long as you don't come off as self-righteous or pompous about your healthy lifestyle, people will be more likely to perceive you as a leader, and thus you are likely to be promoted faster than your overweight or out of shape coworkers. Hundreds of studies prove that fitter, leaner, good looking people get promoted faster and are perceived as more "leader like." [Of course, if you behave like a dumbass, no amount of shredded muscle will help you. You'll still be a dumbass.

Comic book hero

Another cool thing about building a very aesthetically appealing body is that you walk around feeling and looking like a superhero. Superman, or Spiderman, or any of those other comic book characters with amazing bodies… that's you! It's a unique feeling and a major confidence and self-esteem booster.

My theory is that if you know you look your best, you will feel great about that, and you will project a very attractive positive energy that few would ever want to be without. It's an amazing feeling to be able to look in the mirror and see an incredible-looking body. It feels like you got a cheat code for life to enhance your attractiveness. Nothing beats that inner feeling of having your dream body—it's better than having your dream car, your dream vacation, or straight As in college, because you can literally enjoy and experience the benefits of a great body every single second of every single day. A car you can enjoy an hour or two a day. A house you can enjoy a few hours a day. But your body is with you 24/7--you carry it around everywhere you go, and it enhances every second of your life.

If you're after things that truly enhance every aspect of your existence, building a beautiful body is hard to beat. It'll improve how you feel physically, the quality of your relationships, your self esteem, and your social interactions. You'll be perceived as more of an alpha-quality person. Thanks to all that training and regimented eating and discipline, you'll also be able to build a tougher mind. It's a unique and amazing feeling and I would highly recommend anyone to achieve it at least once in their life. Be careful though, because once you have this feeling it's extremely addictive and hard to let go... which is why this next section is particularly important.

Purposeful life and clear direction

Very few things ease the mind better than having a clear direction in life. Knowing who you are and where you need to go in life helps provide that serenity and peace of mind. Building an aesthetically appealing, strong and healthy physique, and really devoting a lot of your time and energy to doing that, can provide you with that direction and purpose. It's also a great way to establish more discipline, structure, and order into your daily and yearly schedule, which will lead to more productivity and less time-wasting doing things that get you nowhere in life.

One of the greatest bonuses I was able to take away from being a lifelong athlete is self-belief. I was confident that I possessed the discipline to see through any goal or dream I had, including completing this book. I always found it a little strange to see people really wanting to achieve something but not having the discipline to achieve it, and quitting when times got tough.

It's a great feeling to trust yourself and know that you can accomplish anything you set your mind to. It's certainly a massive confidence booster. It's a virtuous circle: confidence is the backbone of all success, and successfully pursuing a journey of structure and discipline is a great way of giving that confidence a dramatic and permanent boost.

Money saver

If you're really dedicated to fitness, you probably won't find yourself hitting the bars and clubs 2-3 times a week, throwing away 150-300 bucks a week on alcohol or drugs, or blowing half a paycheck on silly gadgets or trendy going-out clothes. You'll do those things once in a while, but they definitely won't be staple activities. This isn't a universal rule, but for myself at least, I did notice that I saved a tremendous amount of money simply by living a life dedicated to fitness and health.

Functional body

I remember being in Hawaii one time and deciding to swim about a mile out to sea, to a little island I saw in the distance. I hadn't swum that far in years, but knew I could make it to the island, rest there, and swim back whenever I was ready. Before starting on my swim, I was just hanging out a little and taking a look around. I noticed a rather overweight, out-of-shape-looking couple right at the shoreline. They weren't terribly heavy, but clearly showed all the signs of an inactive lifestyle. They were snorkeling in clear water just a foot deep and seemed overly tentative. The water was so clear and shallow you could already see the bottom without any equipment at all, but this was where they felt comfortable putting on goggles and snorkeling. I was blown away by how domesti-cated these people appeared to be. Of course, my observation wasn't really about them in particular—they might have had their reasons for staying so close to shore. But to me they represented the way most people in our society are evolving--no sense of adventure, no useful level of physical fitness, not even suspecting that swimming out to sea, even for 5 minutes, could even be an option. They've spent their entire lives cooped up in houses, in classrooms, and in the office. Stepping out three feet into clear water was already a daunting task full of new adventure for the couple I saw at the beach. I thought how limited their experiences in life must be. I truly felt sorry for them.

If you're fit, you don't have to lead a limited life. You can climb mountains, go on adventures of your liking, go to the beach and look amazing, and most importantly – be proud of the person you see in the mirror.

The best thing is, the more fit you become, the more there will be out there to explore. You're only as limited as your body and mind.

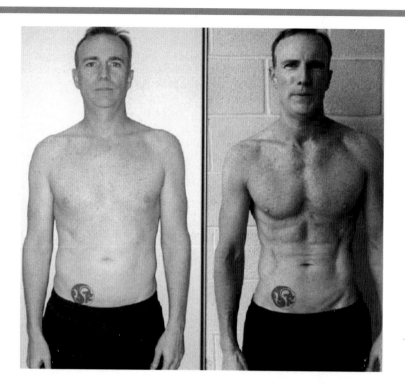

ED McKINNEY

HEALTH-CENTERED LIFESTYLE

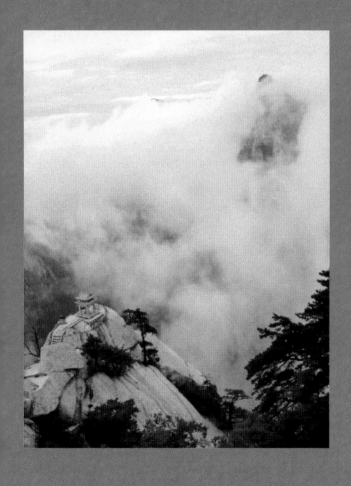

10

The Story Of The Mexican Fisherman Meets Harvard MBA

"A vacationing American businessman standing on the pier of a quaint coastal fishing village in southern Mexico watched as a small boat with just one young Mexican fisherman pulled into the dock. Inside the small boat were several large yellowfin tuna. Enjoying the warmth of the early afternoon sun, the American complimented the Mexican on the quality of his fish.

"How long did it take you to catch them?" the American casually asked.

"Oh, a few hours," the Mexican fisherman replied.

"Why don't you stay out longer and catch more fish?" the American businessman then asked.

The Mexican warmly replied, "With this I have more than enough to support my family's needs."

The businessman then became serious, "But what do you do with the rest of your time?"

Responding with a smile, the Mexican fisherman answered, "I sleep late, play with my children, watch ballgames, and take siesta with my wife. Sometimes in the evenings I take a stroll into the village to see my friends, play the guitar, sing a few songs…"

The American businessman impatiently interrupted, "Look, I have an MBA from Harvard, and I can help you to be more profitable. You can start by fishing several hours longer every day. You can then sell the extra fish you catch. With the extra money, you can buy a bigger boat. With the additional income that larger boat will bring, before long you can buy a second boat, then a third one, and so on, until you have an entire fleet of fishing boats."

Proud of his own sharp thinking, he excitedly elaborated a grand scheme which could bring even bigger profits, "Then, instead of selling your catch to a middleman you'll be able to sell your fish directly to the processor, or even open your own cannery.

Eventually, you could control the product, processing and distribution. You could leave this tiny coastal village and move to Mexico City, or possibly even Los Angeles or New York City, where you could even further expand your enterprise."

Having never thought of such things, the Mexican fisherman asked, "But how long will all this take?"

After a rapid mental calculation, the Harvard MBA pronounced, "Probably about 15-20 years, maybe less if you work really hard."

"And then what, sen or?" asked the fisherman.

"Why, that's the best part!" answered the businessman with a laugh. "When the time is right, you would sell your company stock to the public and become very rich. You would make millions."

"Millions? Really? What would I do with it all?" asked the young fisherman in disbelief.

The businessman boasted, "Then you could happily retire with all the money you've made. You could move to a quaint coastal fishing village where you could sleep late, play with your grandchildren, watch ballgames, and take siesta with your wife. You could stroll to the village in the evenings where you could play the guitar and sing with your friends all you want."
- *Unknown*

I was fortunate enough to study two very intriguing subjects in college: psychology and physiology. Psychology taught me about the human mind, its functions, and its effects on the human body. Physiology, on the other hand, taught me about the body, its functions, and its effects on the human mind. After reading countless books and scientific articles on both subjects, I learned a couple of very important guiding principles, or "laws."

1.   The mind and the body work in tandem. If one is unhealthy, both will become unhealthy. You must attend to the health of the mind as well as the body. It's equally important to have positive thoughts as it is to eat organic food and include dynamic movement in your daily life.

2. We are genetically identical to our hunter-gather ancestors who lived 10,000 years ago. With extremely minor exceptions, there has been no change in our genes for the past 8,000–10,000 years. To optimize your wellbeing, therefore, you need to live the way your body has evolved to live. Physical activity must be embedded in your daily routine. Organic, unprocessed forms of food must be eaten consistently, and stress levels must be managed responsibly.

Studies show that deviating from these basic principles of evolution produces the following pathologies. The further you deviate, the greater the pathology.

1. Physical pathology: Obesity, various skin conditions, accelerated aging, cancer, heart disease, diabetes, and autoimmune disease. Obesity alone is the cause behind 90% of health problems experienced in America. If obesity is eliminated, 90% of the existing health problems in America will disappear. The only way obesity can be eliminated is simply by following the 2nd law described above. Also, remember that the bulk majority of all diseases arise from poor lifestyle and nutritional choices throughout ones life.

2. Psychological lifestyle-induced pathologies: Depression, anxiety, insomnia, lethargy, various panic disorders, dysthymia, anger and frustration problems, and social difficulties. Once again, research shows that one can eliminate most of these issues by simply incorporating the basic principles above consistently.

If our hunter-gatherer ancestors knew how to lead an optimally healthy life, why is it that the average age of death was 35 years of age?

If you factor out deaths from viruses, predators, and accidents, the life expectancy of the hunter-gatherers who lived 10,000 years ago was closer to 60 or 70. Some records even suggest it could have been as much as 90 years of age. Another difference is that a hunter-gatherer at 60 or 70 still had a fully functional body because of a lifetime of physical activity and organic foods, compared to modern day 60 to 70-year-olds who often can't even move around their own house without limitations. Despite the advantages afforded us by the recent boom in medical technology, our hunter-gatherer ancestors were stronger and fitter than we are today. Also, if you take child mortality out of that statistic, people today are only living a few months longer than those who lived 2–3 hundred years ago. And most of that extra time is spent in a nursing home before death. Yes, your heart is beating, but I wouldn't consider that as living. I mentioned this before in the book, but results speak for themselves. Step outside anywhere in America, and 9 out of 10 people you run into are full of mental and physical pain. Full of disease and obesity. Their vitality and soul have long since escaped them.

On top of all that, anthropological research indicates there was no significant incidence of cancer, heart disease, diabetes, or autoimmune disease among our hunter-gather ancestors. On the other hand, half the people in America will experience at least one of the diseases listed above within their lifetime.

Upon graduating from college I was at a crossroads. I could fall into the 9-to-5 office lifestyle like most people do, or I could pursue an alternative lifestyle that focuses on the "laws" presented earlier. I chose the second option, simply because of the following facts:

1. With an office job, I would find myself sitting at a desk 8–10 hours a day, 5 days a week. That type of schedule is completely lacking in physical activity, adventure, and spontaneity. Because of the lack of balance in that lifestyle, I felt certain I would find myself completely burned out on work by the end of year 2. Even if I were passionate about my work, I knew the repetitive nature of my participation in that work would cause me to hate it after a few years. There was no way I'd be able to work for 38 more years with a smile on my face. Also, I felt that type of structure would force me into a mediocre lifestyle because I simply wouldn't have enough time to pursue anything else. I wanted to live my youth to the fullest, because I wasn't going to get another chance to be young.

2. Two weeks' vacation every year was not going to give me enough time to experience true adventure. I knew I would most likely spend those 2 weeks trying to recover mentally from the long hours of work all year. What kind of adventure can you really have in just two weeks, anyway?

3. I most likely would not have enough time or energy to maintain my physical fitness; thus, I would probably gain a lot of weight and age more quickly.

4. If I had a personal goal that needed my full attention, such as finding love or spending more time with that person, I wouldn't be able to focus on it because I would be stuck working Monday through Friday. I would most likely always come home tired and wouldn't really enjoy spending quality time with that person. This applies to various other priorities in life as well.

The basic point I'm trying to make is that the modern-day corporate environment goes against the very basic principles of human evolution. Even if you love what you do, the way that structure makes you do it will cause you to burn out on your work and live an unhealthy lifestyle. When anyone, no matter how passionate, is exposed to one subject frequently enough for too long, that person will get burned out on that subject. It doesn't mean there is something wrong with that person—it's just human nature. For instance, try to remember when you first heard a song that you absolutely loved. It probably made you feel great every time you heard it. However, if you were to keep listening to that song, over and over again, every day, you would begin to habituate to it. At some point, if you continued to listen to that same song for long enough, you might actually begin to hate that song whenever it was played. A similar pattern occurs when people are exposed to the same kind of work for long periods of time, which is exactly what the corporate environment requires.

The modern corporate structure is what is making people unhealthy, and therefore unhappy, simply because that environment ignores basic human evolutionary needs. It's a nasty grind. Understand also that nature is a novelty-generator. Nothing in nature happens twice. Your heart doesn't beat the same way twice; there are no two identical grains of sand, and no two identical leaves on the same tree. Also know that for every single grain of sand there are 20,000 galaxies in space, and for every galaxy there are 100 thousand million stars, and in all that space there is only one you. You're that unique, whether you want to believe it or not—and no corporate environment will ever give you the flexibility to express that uniqueness to its fullest. And because of that, you will grow resentful over time.

If you truly want to live a healthy, well-balanced, adventurous lifestyle - you have to get out of the corporate environment as soon as possible. Being in a corporate environment, with its current structure and form, makes it very difficult for you to live a healthy, balanced lifestyle, especially if you're married and have kids. It's not impossible by any means, but it is near-impossible to sustain over prolonged periods of time. Thus, it would be to your advantage to get out of that type of structure.

Now, the solutions for getting out of a corporate lifestyle are so variable that I cannot reasonably give you personal advice, because I don't know your individual circumstances. However, I can tell you a story about one of my friends:

I had a really smart friend in college. He was super motivated, super smart, and in really good shape throughout our time at school. In fact, he went on to get a masters' degree from an Ivy League school. Once he graduated, he started a job he loved. He worked crazy, long hours, but it was a new job and the projects were a lot of fun. He was always telling me how excited he was about everything, especially the pay.

However, pretty soon the long hours and the stress started to get to him. He gradually stopped working out and stopped pursuing any hobbies, because his work was taking up more and more of his time. Although he was full of energy and excitement in college, he started to become lethargic and generally demotivated. He used to have an adventurous lifestyle, but now he found himself frequenting the same couple of clubs every weekend. He didn't even like clubs, but had no time to pursue other adventures because of his demanding work schedule. His life became mediocre and he began to resent that.

Two years after he started this job he once loved, he often complained about his long hours, lack of work/life balance, inability to find a romantic partner, and his general inability to live life to the fullest. Life was flying by at great speed and he could barely remember an existence that didn't involve sitting behind a desk doing stressful work. However, instead of finding a way out of that lifestyle, he managed to chain himself down even further by buying stuff whenever he got a bonus or promotion. Any extra money he made was spent on expensive purchases that resulted in more bills and more expenses, which only locked him more firmly into a lifestyle he clearly didn't enjoy. He would buy a brand new sports car, or a house, but this provided only a sugar high at best—while at the same time helping solidify his reliance on the very lifestyle he hated.

Nowadays, with so many bills coming in every month, he can't afford to walk away: he has no choice but to continue to work longer and longer hours at a job he clearly stopped liking long ago.

A better strategy, in my opinion, is to continue to strive to make more money (pursuing your meaning in life), but at the same time, aim to decrease your expenses as much as possible. This strategy will give you the luxury of free time which you can use to stay more physically and mentally healthy. It'll also give you the funds you need to pursue an adventurous lifestyle. In addition, you won't have to feel rushed throughout the week or pressed for time. Your stress levels will be tremendously reduced. When you enjoy lower stress levels, you increase the quality of your everyday life experiences tremendously.

Limit leisure costs

I try not to spend a lot of money on my leisure activities unless it involves a cool adventure that's really worth the expenditure. I rarely go to bars or clubs and I rarely spend money on useless stuff. I don't eat out, which helps me save a lot of money all year round. Everything is carefully budgeted, so I end up saving a lot of money that can be used for longer trips, taking continued education courses, and going on adventures instead. This strategy works for me because I don't like bars and clubs anyway. My ideal weekend would include spending time with friends, taking a drive, listening to music, hanging out at a coffee shop, going on an intense hike or mountain climb or hitting the gym. This strategy won't work for everyone, but is worth mentioning. It's certainly effective for those who can incorporate it. Just figure out your core values first and go from there.

Resist social conditioning

Ultimately, the best piece of advice I can give anyone is to follow what's deep inside their heart. Don't pursue a career because it's "safe" or popular. Don't look at what everyone else is doing or wearing or saying. Look at yourself and listen to yourself. Don't be a puppet to social influences and pressures. 9/10 people are sick and miserable anyways. Why follow in their footsteps or try to impressive them? Be yourself and be yourself with confidence. I guarantee you that if people had the freedom to live out their true desires, 90% of people would quit their current job and transition to some other form of work right away. If this is you, why not do it now?

Find a unique job

After college, I decided to become a self-employed personal trainer. I liked the field, I was naturally very good at it, I naturally attracted a lot of clients, and it provided the flexibility and income I desired. My longer term goals are to conduct university-level research, constantly seeking to advance our understanding of health and wellness. Based on my research, I hope to advance the health industry.

Further reading
I would recommend reading and mastering the material in all of the books/programs listed below. I recommend taking notes on each individual book. Write down advice that directly applies to your life and consider how it can be implemented. Then, take rigorous action in implementing that advice and making it work for you.

How to Find and Live Your Legacy DVD series by Paul Chek
If you have trouble identifying who you are, what you want in life, etc. this will be a great start for you. You will not be disappointed with this DVD series

The Law of Success by Napoleon Hill
This book will teach you the character you need to develop to succeed at anything. This text is invaluable, and I would honestly trade my entire college education for the knowledge in this book. Master this material first before moving on to other books.

Rich Dad Poor Dad by Richard Kiyosaki
This book will teach you how people hold themselves back by buying expensive cars, houses, and paying for "higher" education.

4-Hour Work Week by Tim Ferris
This book is unique and will teach you great ways to be more productive with the time you have available. Time efficiency is important and this book will teach you how to master it and to implement a balanced life.

Another thing I like to do is listen to the audio version of these books while I drive. Every single one of these books has a lesson that you can apply immediately to what you're doing in your daily routine in order to enhance the efficiency of that routine. During your morning commute, listen to a single lesson and then practice that lesson all day. Use your life experiences that day to practice those life lessons.

Here is a list of benefits of pursuing what I call the anti-9 to 5 office lifestyle. All of these were done in my first three years after college.
1.   Spent 2 months hiking around China
2.   Spent 2 months living in Japan
3.   Spent 4 month backpacking around India
4.   Spent 2 weeks hiking in Hawaii
5.   Spent 4 weeks hiking in Southern Utah where I got to hike around Angel's Landing, Bryce Canyon, and Antelope Canyon
6.   Climbed Mt. Fury, the long side of Cloud's Rest, and a number of other mountains
7.   Went on a 2 week road trip that ended with spending a week at Burning Man
8.   Went on a 2 week road trip to San Francisco where I got to spend a few nights in Mendocino
9.   Attended countless music festivals and cultural events
10. Stayed in perfect physical shape. I get a full blood panel done every year, and my bloodwork always comes back perfect.
11. Had enough time to draft this book, which was one of my life goals
12. Had enough time to hire a professional dance instructor. I love music, and I always wanted to be a good dancer. With this lifestyle, I was able to become one.
13. Attended acting, improvisation and public speaking classes to overcome a moderate form

of social anxiety I had my entire life. After overcoming that fear, my entire quality of life increased tremendously. I never would have been able to do that under the time constraints of a corporate job. Everyone has something they feel is missing in their life. The great advantage of this type of lifestyle is that you have enough time to fill that void, whether it be a need for more meaningful relationships, longer weekends, or something else.

14. I never feel burned out at work, so I always look forward to going to work.
15. I don't get the feeling that I'm missing out on anything in life. I feel like I'm getting the most I can out of it and living life to the fullest.
16. I look far younger and far healthier than people my age who pursue the 9-to-5 lifestyle.
17. I get to spend quality time with my family and have plenty of "me" time.

On the other hand, here is how my life probably would have looked if I had gone into a 9-to-5, Monday through Friday lifestyle:
1. Work 9-to-5 Monday through Friday
2. Can't do much on the weekends because Saturday and Sunday don't provide enough time to ac-tually go anywhere
3. Work 9-to-5 Monday through Friday
4. Buy an expensive car to justify working these long, stressful hours while I watch my life fly by from behind a desk
5. Gain weight
6. Work 9-to-5 Monday through Friday
7. Gain more weight

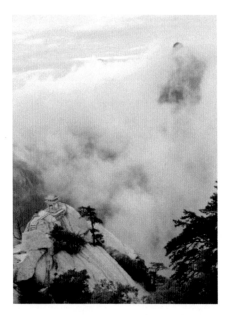

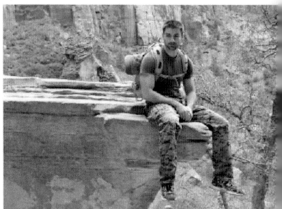

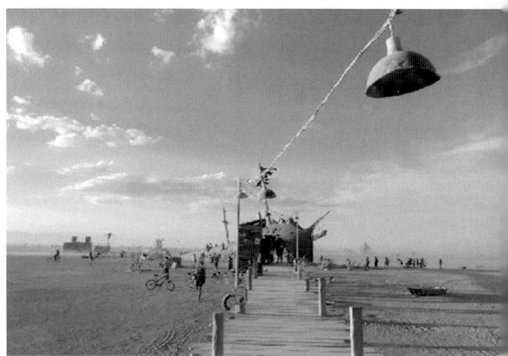

Burning Man 2012

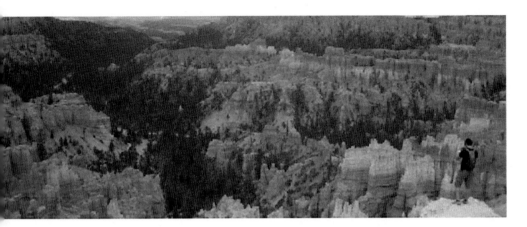

Bryce Canyon 2011

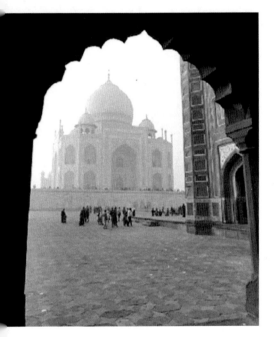

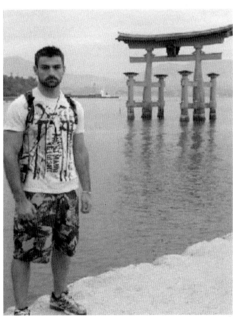

India 2013

Japan 2010

AGELESS SKIN

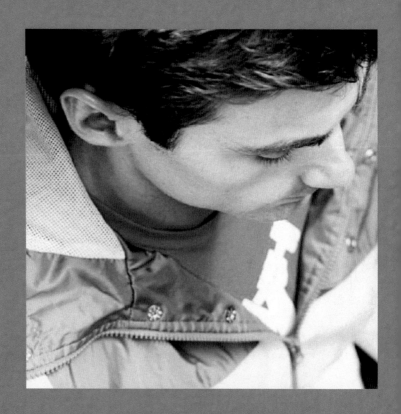

11

Let's start by pointing out that your skin is simply a reflection of what's going on inside your body. If your skin looks bad, it's most likely due to the fact that there is something wrong within your body. Most people in America make the mistake of taking care of their skin from the outside in, mainly relying on creams, face washes, and so on. This is a foolish strategy and will only damage your appearance further.

Here are the steps I personally take to maintain my skin.

Step 1: **5 grams of Omega-3 daily**

I try to get my Omega-3 mainly from real fish, not Omega-3 supplements. Sockeye salmon and sardines are great sources of Omega-3. I also avoid grain-fed meats, which pretty much includes all pork and chicken sold at the supermarket, even if it's organic. For example, even USDA Organic's free-range chicken is vegetarian-fed. And what they mean by vegetarian-fed is that it's grain-fed. It doesn't matter if it's organic—grain is still grain. Chickens are ominvores, not vegetarians. So when an animal is fed an unnatural diet, especially with grains, the Omega-3 goes way down in relation to the Omega-6, which is a pro-inflammatory, and thus a pro-aging, micronutrient. If you find this subject confusing, checkout my book "Anti-Factory Farm Shopping Guide". The book comes with videos to help demystify how to shop for healthy food.

Step 2: **Avoid chemical-laden face washes and creams**

These creams and face washes can actually ruin your skin. Not only do these products age the skin, they also increase the toxic load your body has to endure.

Skin is highly absorbent, and whatever you put on your face is easily absorbed into your blood stream. Most creams, lotions and face washes today have a frightening number of artificial, harmful chemicals in them. These chemicals are absorbed into your body whenever you apply them to your face, increasing your body's total toxic load. When the toxic load becomes heavy enough, your immune system will be weakened and compromised. When the immune system is compromised, your skin starts to look old and unhealthy. Here are the only 2 products I use.

SheaMoisture Jamaican Black Castor Oil Shampoo

Essential Oxygen Certified Organic Toothpaste

If you want to know more about the toxicity of personal care products and other things around us, and learn how to make yourself look younger by decreasing your exposure to hundreds of potentially dangerous chemicals, read the second half of the book Achieving Victory over a Toxic World by Mark Schauss.

Step 3: **Cut out alcohol, drugs, and energy drinks**

This is a big one, especially for women, who are more susceptible than men to the effects of drugs and alcohol. People who drink regularly and use even the smallest amounts of recreational drugs look far more weathered than those who abstain from these substances.

Step 4: **Keep mental stress levels as low as possible**

This is one of the most important factors that determines how fast your skin ages. Mental stress, especially mental stress sustained over long periods of time, has a huge negative impact on the appearance of your skin. Mental stress will age your skin faster than any other factor.

The important thing I feel that needs to be done to lower stress is simply to identify your core values. If you live a life true to those core values, even stressful times won't seem that bad. Real stress happens when people find themselves forced to do things that they don't actually want to be doing. And the worst part is that typically they perceive themselves as being forced, whereas in reality, for example, most people can just walk away from a shitty job. Instead, though, they make up stories to themselves to keep them in that pathological loop of misery. If you struggle in this area, check out *www.journeysofwisdom.com.*

Step 5:   **Watch sugar intake**

Another important determinant of how fast your skin ages is the amount of insulin released into your bloodstream during your lifespan. The more insulin spikes you get, the older you'll look. Here is a list of foods that spike insulin levels. If you're really serious about having picture-perfect skin, it is especially important to avoid "large-spike" category foods.

Large-spike category foods (the worst for your skin) include the following:

1.   Sweets. This includes candy, cake, and just about anything else containing sugar.
2.   Fruit juice. Even if it's organic, it's in your (and your skin's) best interest to avoid it.
3.   Energy drinks and sodas. These will really age your skin. Coca-Cola and Pepsi are probably the worst.
4.   Straight sugar.

Step 6:   **Eat 4–6 cups of raw organic vegetables daily**

This step alone will not only improve your quality of life, but it will also make your skin look amazing. Consuming the quality vitamins and minerals found in vegetables on a regular basis lays the foundation for a stronger immune system. When your immune system is strong, your body is better at fighting off all the illnesses and environmental factors that make your skin look aged and tired. Make sure the vegetables are organic. Nonorganic vegetables have fewer micronutrients and also abundant in trace amounts of synthetic pesticides, fungicides, insecticides and the myriad of other chemicals used to grow factory farmed vegetables. And there is no washing that off. Systmetic pesticides get absorbed into the flesh of the actual crop, so every bit exposes you to trace amounts of these cancer causing chemicals.

Step 7:   **Water**

Another variable I've noticed to have a dramatic impact on the quality of my skin is the amount of water I drink on a daily basis. The more water I drink, the better my skin looks. Water is great at flushing toxins out of your system, and it gives your skin a more hydrated appearance. I try to drink artesian water and drink about half of my body weight in ounces daily. So if I'm 200lbs, I would strive to drink 100 ounces daily.

Step 8:   **Sun exposure**

Contrary to what most people believe, moderate sun exposure on a weekly basis not only strengthens your immune system and gives you more energy throughout the week, but it also makes your skin look better. When the weather permits, I try to allow 25 to 30 minutes of exposure every Wednesday and Sunday. I try to spend an equal amount of time sunning my body from all sides. Also, I generally cover my entire face with a thick towel or shirt. You want to avoid using sunscreen during your sunning sessions because the sunscreen will hinder Vitamin D3 absorption, which is the whole reason for sun exposure.

Step 9:   **Steam room**

Blackheads cause breakouts, and steam is great for clearing blackheads from facial and body skin alike. In the hot environment of a steam room, your body is fooled into reacting as if you were sick, so it releases natural anti-oxidants. Anti-oxidants have numerous health benefits, including making your skin look better. Naturally, you will need to bring a lot of water to drink. I try to hit the steam room once a week for about 20-30 minutes. However, if you're new to it, you'll probably only last 2-5 minutes at first. For beginners, I would recommend going in and out of the steam room at desired intervals. I only wear shorts and sandals when using the steam room.

The 9 steps outlined above serve as a foundation for perfect skin. If you take these measures consistently, I promise you will have better looking skin and you will look younger, for longer. Once again, however, they need to be implemented very consistently to be truly effective.

In addition to the steps above, there are other measures you can take to perfect your skin and overall well-being.

Bath

Once a week, I go through the following routine. I usually do this every Sunday night since it helps my skin look better, but also serves as a de-stressing activity that helps me get ready for the week ahead. I use Epsom salts and keep a gallon of iced water to drink right next to the bath tub. I also keep a small towel accessible for step #8.

First, I run a bath. I try to use fairly hot water, because heat helps open the pores of the skin, which makes it easier to cleanse the skin. The bath usually takes 15-20 minutes to fill, which leaves time for the following steps:

1. Trim nose hair.
2. Clip nails.
3. By now the bath is ready. I usually soak for about 30-45 minutes and practice just focusing on my breathing. I usually place a warm towel over my face.

Body hair and shaving

Body hair can look good on some guys, but large quantities of body hair also hide muscle definition and striations. If you want to look as defined as possible, having little to no body hair is preferable. However, I wouldn't recommend shaving too frequently for most of the body. It's better to use an electric shaver, such as Wahl's 9854-500 Electric Shaver, and just trim your hair once a week or so. Ideally, you want to use the lowest setting possible.

For arms, however, it's worth it to shave every other day, because it's quick and really enhances muscle definition.

A few tips to get the best possible shave:

Fill a small cup with very hot water, and place your shaver in the cup. Let the shaver sit in the cup for about 10 minutes before starting to shave.

If possible, plan to shave while taking a hot shower. This will always provide a better result than shaving near the sink in a cooler environment. I prefer to stand in a warm shower for about 5 minutes before I begin to shave. This allows the pores to loosen up, ensuring a much better shave.

I prefer to use a Gillette Fusion Brand Razor and try to change the blade every other week. For shaving cream, I recommend Aveeno's Therapeutic Shave Gel.

The perfect tan

A good tan can really help increase your aesthetic appeal by improving the appearance of your skin. A tan also helps you look more defined and muscular, especially around the midsection. There are several ways to achieve a good tan, but I generally don't use tanning beds. Not only are they unsafe and skin-damaging, but in my experience they can also be quite dirty, and I've noticed minimal results with them.

Spray tan

Spray tans are great, because you can achieve a perfect tan in about 3 minutes. I usually don't use self-tanners at home because I find them more difficult to apply evenly over the entire body, especially the back. Instead, I just go to a tanning salon. I always select a personalized tan option, which runs about 30 to 40 dollars in my area. This type of tan will last about 2 weeks, depending on your bathing habits, whether or not you use scrubs and exfoliants, and so on. The tan always looks perfect and very natural. This is an especially good option for those who burn easily or simply do not tan naturally. You only really need to do this when you want the muscles to really show for a photoshoot or something like that. You wouldn't want to do this on a regular basis.

Pearly-white smiles and dental care

Perfectly white teeth also add to your overall aesthetic appeal. If your teeth are just not naturally white, and don't seem improve no matter how much you brush, I recommend getting a whitening procedure done at your dentist's office. I had this procedure done a long time ago, and it has been very effective in whitening my teeth and keeping them that way for years, even without touch-ups. It's an affordable procedure for most people, and my confidence certainly soared knowing that every time I smiled my teeth looked really white. I would highly recommend the procedure to anyone seeking a beautiful smile.

In terms of general dental care, you should brush at least twice daily: once in the morning and once at night. I use an electric toothbrush, which I consider a good investment in my health and dental care. I use Philips Sonicare Elite HX6911. Try to make sure your brand of toothpaste is organic—there are so many chemicals in most brands of toothpaste.

I always found flossing annoying until I purchased a Comfort Clean Flosser from Den Tek. This made flossing much easier, and after I started using it I became far more consistent about flossing. You should aim to floss at least once a day.

Mouthwash is also another tool you can use to increase your appeal. No one likes bad breath, and rinsing consistently can keep bad breath at bay. I rinse once every morning.

Body odor

If you want to present yourself to the world in the best possible light, it's very important to make sure you have body odor under control. Body odor can make anyone repulsive, even if you're physically attractive. I personally use Crystal Deodorant Stick, which is chemical free and unscented.

Cocoa butter for stretch marks

Cocoa butter with vitamin E is a great way to prevent stretch marks. Make sure to purchase a cream formulation rather than lotion, which is less effective. For best results, you will want to use cocoa butter twice weekly. Make sure to rub it thoroughly into the affected area. Typical areas to check for stretch marks are the chest, front shoulders, biceps, and all around the lower midsection. I like to use Palmer-s Cocoa Butter Formula with Vitamin E.

Hair

Having a good haircut that fits your personal style and compliments your physical features is very important and will really work to your advantage when seeking to enhance your aesthetic appeal. One of the best ways to find the haircut that suits you best is to experiment-- try a variety of different haircuts and different hairstylists. You can even try different colors. Find the one style that you're 100% comfortable with, the one that really raises your confidence level. If you don't trust your own artistic instincts, simply ask someone whose opinion you respect and follow their advice.

For hair products, I love Enjoy's Dry Wax. It leaves your hair looking natural and not "gelled up." I generally apply the product when my hair is almost, but not completely dry. It provides a fairly strong hold so your hairstyle won't fall apart an hour later.

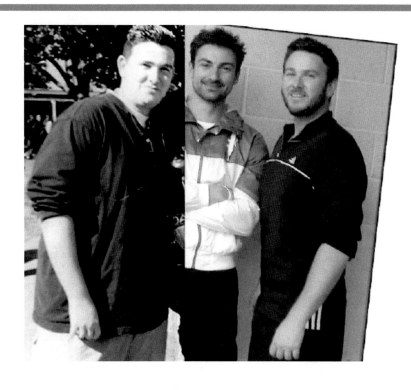

SEAN GORGIE

PERFECT POSTURE

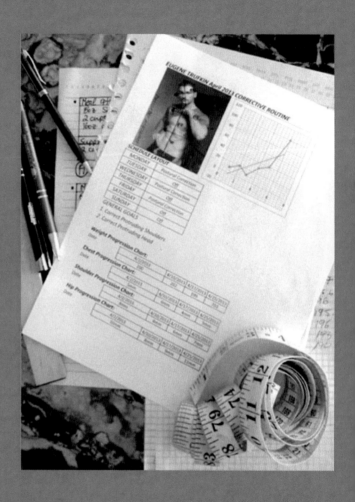

12

Very few people realize this, but you can easily make your midsection look 1 to 1.5 inches smaller just by standing with perfect posture instead of slumping.

Another advantage of perfect posture is that it makes your muscles look longer and leaner and makes you appear taller, all of which are attractive traits. In addition, a person who has perfect posture will always appear far more confident than one who slouches all day.

Below you will find a list of the most common postural problems which can make your midsection look bigger and make you appear shorter. This section also covers the reasons behind postural problems, and how to go about fixing them.

Note: Any postural problem is the result of a group of muscles that are too tight and a group of muscles that are too weak. To correct the postural problem, you have to strengthen the weak muscles and loosen up the tight muscles. To have long lasting change, you must avoid sitting for multiple hours daily. No amount of working out and stretching will be able to offset the damage sitting for 8-10 hours a day does to your body. If good posture is something that's important for you, you must avoid sitting all day. Even a few hours daily really messes you up tremendously.

Protruding shoulders

Muscles that are too tight: subscapularis, all anterior rotators of the shoulder, lats, rectus abdominis, pectoralis majorand minor, and biceps. Solution: You have to massage out and stretch out these muscles.
Muscles that are too weak: Muscles that are too weak: posterior shoulder, rhomboids, thoracic extensors, external rotators, lower and mid/lower traps, and cervical flexors. **Solution:** You have to strengthen these muscles.

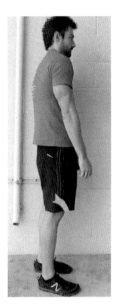

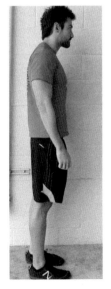

Protruding head

Muscles that are too tight: subscapularis, all anterior rotators of the shoulder, latissimus dorsi, rectus abdominis, pectoralis major and minor, biceps, anterior, medial, and posterior scalene, upper traps, sternocleidomastoid, and levator scapulae. **Solution:** You have to massage out and stretch out these muscles.

Front hip tilt

Muscles that are too tight: lumbar erectors, quads, and psoas. **Solution:** You have to massage out and stretch out these muscles.

Muscles that are too weak: gluteus maximus, hamstrings, and lower abs. **Solution:** You have to strengthen these muscles.

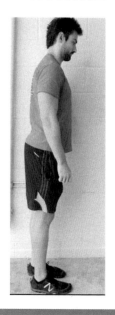

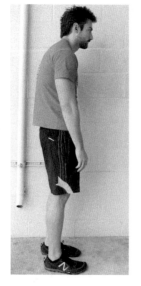

Slouching

Muscles that are too tight: subscapularis, all anterior rotators of the shoulder, lats, rectus abdominis, pectoralis major and minor, biceps, anterior, medial, and posterior scalene, upper traps, sternocleidomastoid, levator scapulae, gluteus maximus, and hamstrings. **Solution:** You have to massage out and stretch out these muscles.

Muscles that are too weak: posterior shoulder, rhomboids, thoracic extensors, external rotators, lower and mid traps, cervical flexors, thoracic extensors, and lower abs. **Solution:** You have to strengthen these muscles.

Other benefits of postural correction

Another great benefit of having your body's musculature restored to its proper alignment is that you'll experience significantly less pain throughout your body, because muscles will fall into natural alignment. With perfect posture, your muscles won't be forced to operate at unnatural angles which can cause prolonged strain and pain. 90% of cases of back pain and general back problems could easily be annihilated if the affected people were able to achieve perfect posture. Imagine that! No more back pain and no surgery needed--and you get to have perfect posture, look taller, look leaner, and just generally appear more badass. At the end of the day, you really do have to strive to avoid sitting for many hours daily. This is your only hope at achieving better posture.

Other lifestyle tips to enhance your posture

Lose the oversized pillow

Many people sleep on pillows which are far too thick. The pillow forces their head up at an extreme angle throughout the entire night. Ideally, your head should be perfectly aligned with your spine, not tilted up at an angle.

If you work at a desk, this problem is compounded. You spend all day sitting with your head protruded forward, then if you sleep on your back, you go home and sleep all night with your head protruded forward. These continuous patterns cause your head to adopt this angle habitually and stay that way, resulting in poor posture.

It's easy to eliminate this problem. Simply switch to a thinner pillow or stop using a pillow at all, and implement the postural exercises listed above.

Use a computer screen stand and make sure it's aligned with your gaze

Another great way to fix your posture is to make sure your computer screen at work is positioned directly in front of your face, on an elevated surface. It should be elevated enough to ensure that it feels more natural to sit straight than it does to hunch over. If you combine this tactic with the pillow tactic described above, you should notice a good improvement in your posture, which will be accompanied by less stiffness and pain in the neck and upper back. Although it's not that much better than sitting, try to get a standing desk. This is a good move in the right direction.

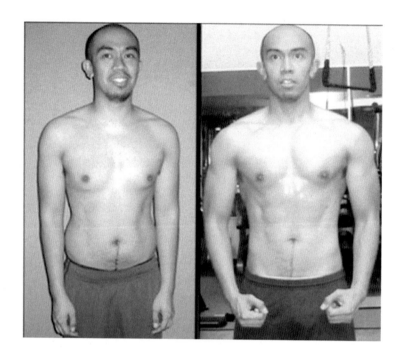

CHUCK RABINA

EVGENY
TRUFKIN

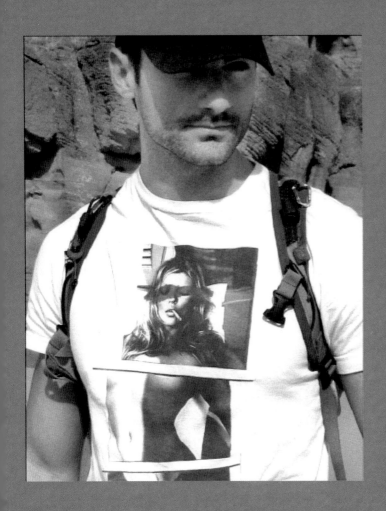

13

ACADEMIC AWARDS:

- Latin Honors Gold Cord recipient
- Academic Presidential Distinction Award
- Golden Key International Academic Honor recipient
- The National Honor Society in Psychology Academic recipient
- Dean's Honor List at U.C.I.

CERTIFICATIONS:

- Bachelors in Psychology from UCI (3.7/4.0 GPA)
- National Academy of Sports Medicine Graduate
- CHEK Institute Trained Professional (HLC1/HLC2 Certified)
- Apex Certified Trainer
- CPR Certified

Other:
- Author of «Laws of Aesthetics» and « Anti-Factory Farm Shopping Guide»
- Fat Loss Lecturer at Disneyland, US Army Reserve Center, and Sealy

2013

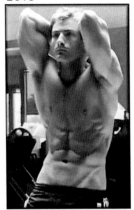

2012

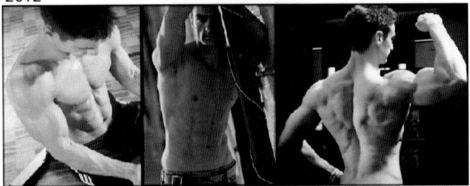

2010

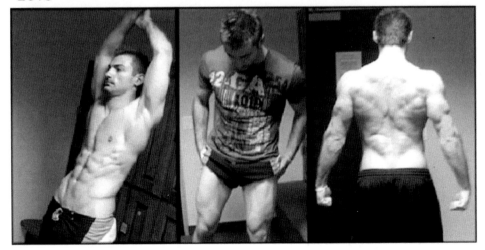

2005

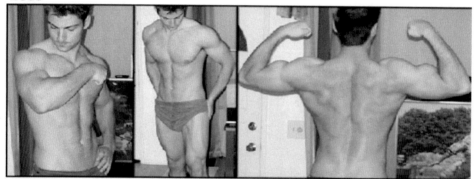

2003

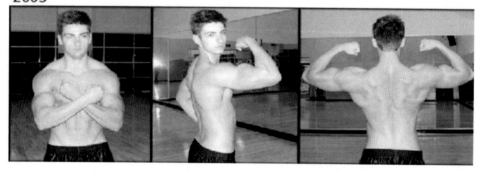

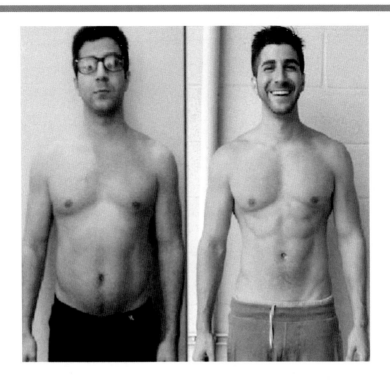

ARMEN AVAKIAN

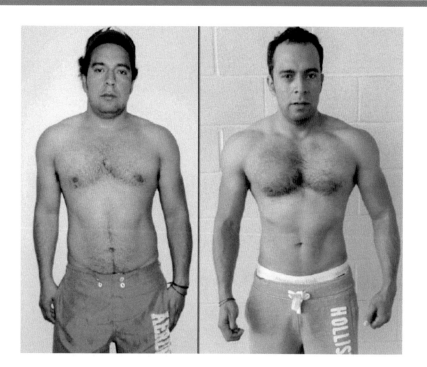

CARLOS DORADO

Made in the USA
Columbia, SC
02 November 2019